ADRENAL FATIGUE RELIEF DIET COOKBOOK:

Revitalize Your Energy, Restore Your Vitality

Dr. Vera J. Reynolds

Copyright

This book is a work of non-fiction. The information, opinions, and advice presented in this book are based on the author's research and personal experience. The author and publisher make no representation or warranties with respect to the accuracy or completeness of the contents of this book and specifically disclaim any implied warranties of merchantability or fitness for a particular purpose.

The information contained in this book is provided on an "as is" basis and is intended to be used for general informational purposes only. The views and opinions expressed in this book are those of the author and do not necessarily reflect the official policy or position of any agency, organization, employer, or company.

Contents

INTRODUCTION

In the frenzy of contemporary life, our bodies frequently carry the brunt of stress, leaving us feeling drained and exhausted. But worry not, because inside the "Adrenal Fatigue Relief Diet Cookbook pages," a revolutionary culinary trip awaits—a voyage that promises to revive your energy, restore your vitality, and kindle a newfound feeling of health. Prepare to embark on a tour via healthy dishes expertly designed to support your adrenal health and pave the road to a bright and happy existence.

A Symphony of Flavor and Wellness

The "Adrenal Fatigue Relief Diet Cookbook" is not simply a collection of recipes—it's a symphony of tastes, textures, and nutrients that meet the unique requirements of those looking to overcome adrenal fatigue. Rooted in holistic health, this cookbook encourages you to discover the harmonious interplay of foods nourishing your body and spirit.

From the earliest crack of morning to the twilight hours, each dish inside these pages has been thoughtfully designed to balance healing and enjoyment. Whether you are a culinary newbie or a seasoned chef, our cookbook lets you take care of your wellness through mindful eating.

Your Passport to Revitalization

Imagine waking up each morning feeling rejuvenated and ready to confront the day ahead. Picture yourself eating meals that excite your taste senses and supply the sustenance your body wants. The "Adrenal Fatigue Relief Diet Cookbook" serves as your passport to regeneration, leading you through a thorough culinary experience to ease tiredness, reduce stress, and build a deeper connection with your body's intrinsic knowledge.

A Feast for the Senses

Prepare to pamper your senses as you immerse yourself in a treasure trove of dishes spanning gourmet bliss. From the vivid colours of nutrient-packed smoothie bowls to the soothing fragrances drifting from a boiling pot of substantial stew, this cookbook appeals to your senses in ways that nurture your body and soul.

The Blueprint for Optimal Adrenal Health

With the "Adrenal Fatigue Relief Diet Cookbook" in your hands, you possess the blueprint for maximum adrenal health. Dive into chapters with breakfast boosters that jumpstart your day with prolonged energy. Explore nourishing foods that quiet those noon cravings while supporting your adrenals. Discover healthful lunches and meals that make each mouthful a step toward regeneration.

More Than a Cookbook

Beyond its position as a cookbook, this literary gem offers a guide to comprehending the fundamental relationship between our foods and our total health. Delve into sections that clarify the complicated network of adrenal health, bringing insights into the significance of diet, stress management, and mindful eating.

Embrace the Culinary Renaissance

The "Adrenal Fatigue Relief Diet Cookbook" heralds a culinary renaissance that embraces the marriage of food and enjoyment. Let go of the illusion that nutritious eating requires sacrifice because, inside these pages, you'll learn the skill of producing tasty and helpful meals.

Your Invitation to Wellness

Are you ready to grab the reins of your health journey? The "Adrenal Fatigue Relief Diet Cookbook" invites embracing wellbeing in all aspects. From the rewarding delight of making meals that respect your body's demands to the joy of indulging in tastes that energize your senses, this cookbook provides a route to sustainable change.

Elevate Your Wellbeing, One Recipe at a Time

Step into the realm of the "Adrenal Fatigue Relief Diet Cookbook" and start on an adventure toward increased health. Let the pages guide you as you construct meals that nourish, heal, and spark your inner energy. With each dish, you are regaining your vitality and embracing the power of self-care.

So, whether you want to overcome adrenal fatigue, increase your energy levels, or delight in the pleasure of vivid food, the "Adrenal

Fatigue Relief Diet Cookbook" is your ultimate companion on the path to regained health, balance, and resilience. Open its pages, relish its aromas, and allow it to be your beacon of inspiration as you traverse the road toward maximum health.

CHAPTER ONE

Understanding Adrenal Fatigue

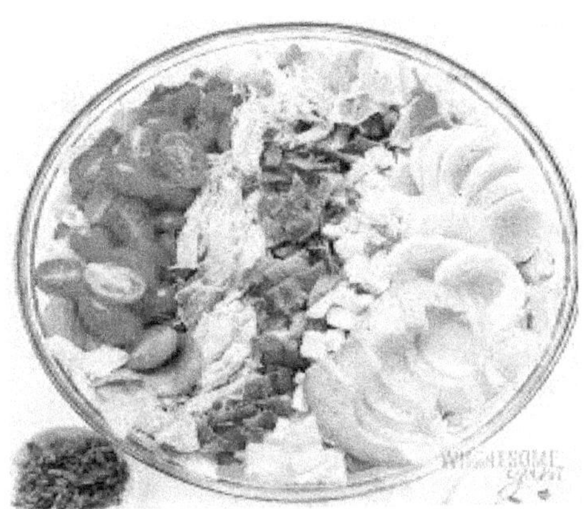

Adrenal fatigue is a word used to describe a condition of imbalance in the body induced by continuous periods of stress and its influence on the adrenal glands. These little, pyramid-shaped glands on each kidney are crucial in regulating different biological activities, including stress response, metabolism, immune system support, and energy generation.

1. **Adrenal Gland Function:** The adrenal glands generate numerous vital hormones, with cortisol being one of the most well-known. Cortisol helps your body adapt to stress by boosting blood sugar levels, inhibiting the immune system momentarily, and controlling inflammation. Adrenaline, another hormone generated by these glands, activates the "fight or flight" response in circumstances of extreme stress.

2. **Symptoms of Adrenal Fatigue:** When the adrenal glands are repeatedly stimulated owing to prolonged stress, they may become overworked and less effective in generating hormones. This may lead to several symptoms, such as:

3. **Persistent Fatigue:** Feeling fatigued even after a whole night's sleep.
4. **Sleep Disturbances:** Difficulty falling asleep or remaining asleep during the night.

5. **Weight Fluctuations:** Unexplained weight gain or loss, typically accompanied by cravings for unhealthy foods.

6. **Mood Changes:** Increased irritation, anxiety, and even melancholy.

7. **Digestive Issues:** Problems including bloating, constipation, or diarrhoea.

8. **Low Energy Levels:** A need for more energy, particularly in the morning or throughout the day.

9. **Difficulty Concentrating:** Inability to concentrate or recall things.

Causes and Triggers:

Chronic stress is a primary factor in adrenal exhaustion. Other things that might initiate or worsen this illness include:

1. **Work Pressure:** Long hours, high expectations, and deadlines.
2. **Emotional Stress:** Relationship concerns, financial anxieties, and personal problems.
3. **Lifestyle Choices:** Poor nutrition, lack of exercise, excessive coffee or sugar consumption, and inadequate sleep.
4. **Environmental Factors:** Exposure to poisons and contaminants.

Controversy and Diagnosis:

It's crucial to remember that not all medical practitioners acknowledge adrenal exhaustion as a unique medical problem. Symptoms of adrenal fatigue overlap with those of other health concerns, making it tough to diagnose. If you have adrenal fatigue, visit a healthcare physician to avoid further problems and obtain appropriate assistance.

Influence on wellness: Adrenal fatigue isn't just about feeling tired; it may substantially impact your health. It may damage your immune system, making you more prone to infections. It may also interfere with your capacity to handle stress efficiently and maintain emotional equilibrium.

Comprehensive strategy: Addressing adrenal fatigue demands a comprehensive approach that spans all parts of your life. In the future chapters of this book, we will examine how diet, stress management strategies, and lifestyle changes may help ease adrenal exhaustion and restore balance to your body.

By knowing the underlying mechanics of adrenal fatigue and its consequences on your body, you'll be more able to make educated decisions that support your path toward higher energy levels, more excellent mood, and overall well-being.

Importance of Nutrition in Recovery

Nutrition plays a crucial part in the healing process from adrenal exhaustion. What you consume immediately affects your adrenal glands, hormonal balance, and general wellness. This chapter will examine how particular nutrients and dietary choices assist your body's healing process.

1. **Balancing Blood Sugar Levels:** Stabilizing blood sugar levels is vital for controlling adrenal exhaustion. Consuming complex carbs like whole grains, veggies, and legumes helps minimize energy dumps and provides constant energy throughout the day.

2. **Anti-Inflammatory Foods:** Chronic stress may contribute to inflammation in the body, aggravating adrenal exhaustion symptoms. Incorporating anti-inflammatory foods such as leafy greens, berries, oily salmon, and turmeric will help decrease inflammation and improve healing.

3. **Adrenal-Supportive Nutrients:** Certain nutrients are beneficial for adrenal health. These include:

- **Vitamin C:** Found in citrus fruits, bell peppers, and strawberries, it improves adrenal gland function and helps control stress.
- **B Vitamins:** Essential for energy generation and stress control. Sources include whole grains, leafy vegetables, and lean meats.
- **Magnesium:** Supports relaxation and stress reduction. Nuts, seeds, and leafy greens are excellent sources.
- **Zinc:** Important for immune function and hormone control. It is found in lean meats, nuts, and legumes.
- **Healthy Fats:** Including healthy fats from sources like avocados, nuts, seeds, and olive oil will assist hormone synthesis and help maintain steady energy levels.

4. **Hydration:** Staying well-hydrated helps the body's stress response and general performance. Herbal teas, infused water, and ingesting water-rich foods aid in hydration.

5. **Avoiding Trigger Meals:** Certain meals might aggravate adrenal fatigue symptoms. Limit or avoid caffeine, refined sweets, processed meals, and excessive salt since these may stress the adrenals and disturb hormonal balance.

6. **Regular Meals and Snacking:** Regularly eating balanced meals and snacks helps reduce blood sugar spikes and crashes, maintaining sustainable energy levels.

7. **Mindful Eating:** Practicing mindful eating helps alleviate stress on the body. Slow down, appreciate your meals, and heed your body's hunger and fullness signals.

8. **Meal Planning for Recovery:** Creating well-rounded meals that contain complex carbs, lean proteins, healthy fats, and a range of colourful veggies is crucial to supplying your body with the resources it needs.

9. **Individualized Approach:** It's crucial to remember that each person's dietary demands are unique. Consulting a healthcare expert or registered dietitian specializing in adrenal health may help you customize your diet to your needs.

Adopting a balanced and nutrient-rich diet may support your body's healing process, increase your energy levels, and reduce the symptoms of adrenal fatigue. The recipes and meal planning in the subsequent chapters will give practical methods to put these concepts into action and boost your general wellness.

CHAPTER TWO

The Basics of Adrenal-Friendly Cooking

Building a Balanced Plate

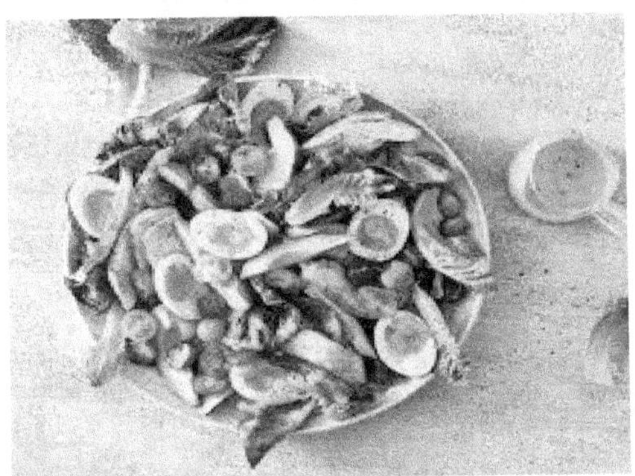

Creating a balanced plate is a cornerstone of aiding your body's recovery from adrenal exhaustion. In this chapter, you'll discover how to plan meals to deliver essential nutrients, control blood sugar levels, and encourage healthy adrenal function.

The Components of a Balanced Plate:

1. **Quality Protein Source:** Include lean proteins such as fowl, fish, tofu, beans, or lentils. Protein helps muscle regeneration, hormone synthesis, and sustained energy.

2. **Complex Carbohydrates:** Opt for whole grains like quinoa, brown rice, or whole wheat pasta. These give a consistent supply of energy and minimize blood sugar rises.

3. **Healthy Fats:** Incorporate sources, including avocados, nuts, seeds, and olive oil. Healthy fats help in hormone production and enhance overall well-being.

4. **Colourful veggies:** Fill half your plate with a variety of veggies. Different hues signify distinct nutrients that help with immune health, digestion, and antioxidant support.

5. **Fiber-Rich Foods:** Whole grains, veggies, and legumes contain fibre that aids digestion and helps maintain stable blood sugar levels.

Portion Control and Proportions:

- **Protein:** Aim for a portion roughly the size of your hand. This guarantees appropriate protein intake without overwhelming your dish.
- **Carbs:** Fill a quarter of your plate with complex carbs like healthy grains or starchy veggies.
- **Veggies:** Allocate half your plate to veggies, emphasizing variety and colour.
- **Fats:** Include a modest portion of healthy fats, such as a sprinkle of almonds or a drizzle of olive oil.

Enhancing Nutrient Density:

- **Leafy Greens:** Incorporate nutrient-rich greens like spinach, kale, or Swiss chard for vitamins and minerals.
- **Colour Variety:** Choose a variety of coloured veggies to provide a broad spectrum of antioxidants and phytonutrients.

- **Herbs and Spices:** Flavor your meals with herbs and spices like turmeric, ginger, and garlic, which give both flavour and health benefits.

Meal Examples:

Grilled Chicken Plate:
- Grilled chicken breast (protein)
- Quinoa (complex carbohydrate)
- Steamed broccoli and carrots (colourful veggies)
- Drizzle of olive oil (healthy fat)

Tofu Stir-Fry:
- Tofu cubes stir-fried with mixed veggies (protein)
- Brown rice (complex carbohydrate)
- Sautéed spinach and bell peppers (colourful veggies)
- Sesame seeds sprinkled on top (healthy fat)

Balanced Snacking:
- Apply the same concepts to your snacks by incorporating a protein source (e.g., Greek yoghurt, hummus), carbohydrate (e.g., whole-grain crackers, fruit), and some vegetables.

By generating balanced plates, you'll feed your body with the nutrients it needs to heal from adrenal exhaustion, normalize energy levels, and maintain overall wellness. The recipes and meal ideas in the following chapters will help you put this information into effect for tasty and wholesome dinners.

Optimal adrenal health relies on a spectrum of critical nutrients that promote hormone synthesis, stress response, and general wellness. In this chapter, we'll look into essential nutrients that significantly maintain good adrenal function.

1. **Vitamin C:** Vitamin C is a potent antioxidant that helps resist stress and promotes adrenal gland function. It's crucial for manufacturing cortisol and other stress-related chemicals. Citrus fruits, bell peppers, strawberries, and broccoli are rich suppliers.

2. **B Vitamins:** B vitamins, notably B5 (pantothenic acid), generate adrenal hormones and energy metabolism. B6 and B12 are also vital for mood modulation and nerve function. Whole grains, lean meats, fish, eggs, and leafy greens are rich in B vitamins.

3. Magnesium is regarded as the "relaxation mineral" crucial for reducing stress and fostering relaxation. It enhances muscular function, sleep quality, and general stress reduction. Nuts, seeds, whole grains, and leafy greens are excellent sources.

4. Zinc is vital for immune function, hormone balance, and wound healing. It helps regulate cortisol levels and improves overall adrenal health. You may get zinc in lean meats, nuts, seeds, and legumes.

5. **Omega-3 Fatty Acids:** Omega-3s have anti-inflammatory qualities and improve brain function. They

have a role in modulating stress response and mood. Fatty fish (such as salmon and sardines), flaxseeds, chia seeds, and walnuts are excellent sources.

6. **Adaptogens:** While not nutrients in the classic sense, adaptogenic herbs like ashwagandha, Rhodiola, and holy basil have been demonstrated to assist the body in adapting to stress and maintaining adrenal balance.

7. **Protein:** Adequate protein consumption is needed for hormone synthesis, muscle repair, and general energy. Including lean protein sources like chicken, fish, tofu, and lentils in your diet helps adrenal function.

8. **Iron:** Iron is essential for oxygen transfer and energy synthesis. Iron deficiency may contribute to exhaustion and aggravate adrenal fatigue symptoms. Include iron-rich foods like lean meats, beans, lentils, and spinach.

9. **Antioxidants:** Antioxidants in colourful fruits and vegetables help protect cells from oxidative damage produced by chronic stress and inflammation.

10. **Hydration:** Staying hydrated promotes adrenal function and helps regulate stress. Herbal teas and infused water may help with both hydration and nutritional intake.

11. **Probiotics:** A healthy gut is connected to general wellness, including stress control. Probiotic-rich foods like yoghurt and fermented foods boost intestinal health.

12. **Individualized Approach:** Every individual's dietary demands are unique. Consulting a healthcare physician or certified dietitian may help you understand which nutrients are necessary for your body's recovery.

By including these critical nutrients in your diet, you'll be taking strides toward supporting your adrenal function and encouraging overall well-being. The recipes and meal ideas in the subsequent chapters will help you build healthful meals that focus on these nutrients.

CHAPTER THREE

Breakfast Boosters

Chia Seed Yogurt Parfait

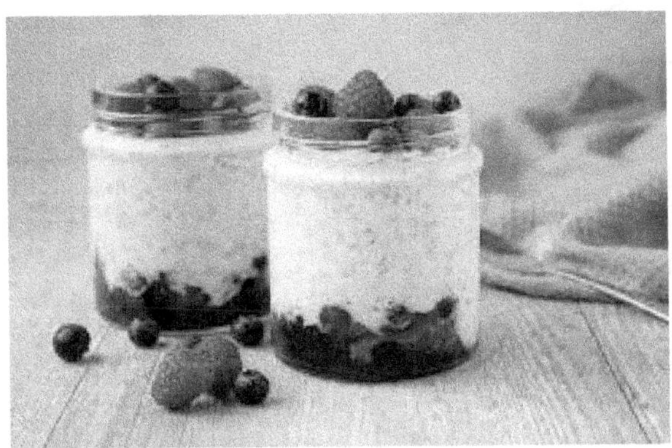

Ingredients:

- Greek yoghurt (unsweetened)
- Chia seeds
- Mixed berries (e.g., strawberries, blueberries, raspberries)
- Honey or maple syrup (optional for sweetness)
- Nuts or seeds (e.g., almonds, walnuts, sunflower seeds)
- Granola (optional, for crunch)

Instructions:

1. **Prepare the Chia Seed Pudding:**
   - Combine two teaspoons of chia seeds in a small dish or glass with roughly 1/2 cup of Greek yoghurt.
   - Stir well to blend and ensure the chia seeds are uniformly distributed.

2. **Let It Set:**
   - Cover the bowl or glass and chill the mixture for at least 2-3 hours or overnight. The chia seeds will absorb the yoghurt and thicken the mix during this time.

3. **Assemble the Parfait:**
   - Grab a serving glass or bowl once the chia seed pudding has been set.
   - Start by putting a scoop of chia seed pudding at the bottom.

4. **Add Berries:**
   - Add a layer of mixed berries on top of the chia seed pudding. You may use a mix of sliced strawberries, blueberries, and raspberries.

5. **Repeat Layers:**
   - Add another layer of chia seed pudding on top of the fruit.
   - Add another layer of mixed berries on top of the chia seed pudding.

6. **Top with Nuts and Sweetener:**
    - Sprinkle a handful of chopped nuts or seeds atop the berry layer for extra crunch and nutrients.
    - If you desire more sweetness, sprinkle a tiny quantity of honey or maple syrup over the top.

7. **Optional Granola Layer:**
    - If you prefer, put a layer of granola on top for an added layer of texture and taste.

8. **Serve and Enjoy:**
    - Your Chia Seed Yogurt Parfait is ready to be enjoyed! Use a big spoon to scoop each layer for a delightful and healthy breakfast.

This Chia Seed Yogurt Parfait is high in protein, fibre, healthy fats, and antioxidants, making it a fantastic option to start your day with sustained energy and support for adrenal health. Feel free to alter the ingredients and amounts depending on your tastes and dietary requirements.

Sweet Potato Toast

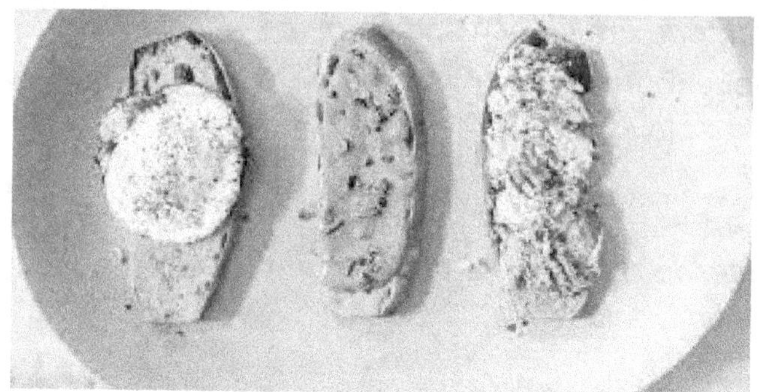

Ingredients:

- Medium-sized sweet potato
- Toppings of your choosing (see choices below)

Instructions:

1. **Slice the Sweet Potato:**

- Wash and peel the sweet potato.
- Slice the sweet potato lengthwise into thin, even slices, approximately ¼ to ½ inch thick. These pieces will act as your "toast."

2. **Toaster Method:**
- Preheat your toaster in the highest setting.
- Place the sweet potato slices in the toaster and toast them for a few cycles until they are cooked and slightly

crispy around the edges. The precise time will depend on your toaster, so keep an eye on them.

3. **Oven Method:**
   - Preheat your oven to 375°F (190°C).
   - Place the sweet potato slices on a baking sheet lined with parchment paper. You may delicately brush the slices with olive oil if desired.
   - Bake in the oven for approximately 15-20 minutes, rotating the slices halfway through until they are cooked and somewhat crispy.

4. **Top with Toppings:**
   - Once your sweet potato toasts are done, it's time to add toppings!
   - Here are a few topping options to consider:
   - Avocado slices and poached egg
   - Almond butter and banana slices
   - Greek yoghurt with mixed fruit
   - Cottage cheese with sliced strawberries
   - Hummus and sliced cucumber or tomato
   - Ricotta cheese and honey drizzle
   - Smoked salmon with cream cheese
   - Sautéed spinach with feta cheese

5. **Season and Enjoy:**
   - Sprinkle your selected toppings with a bit of salt, pepper, or any spices of your choosing.

- Enjoy your Sweet Potato Toast creation!

This Sweet Potato Toast is an excellent source of complex carbs, dietary fibre, and other nutrients. It's a flexible basis for several toppings that may offer a well-rounded and healthy breakfast to boost your adrenal health and energy levels. Feel free to be creative with your toppings and personalize this recipe to your taste preferences.

Spinach and Mushroom Frittata Recipe:

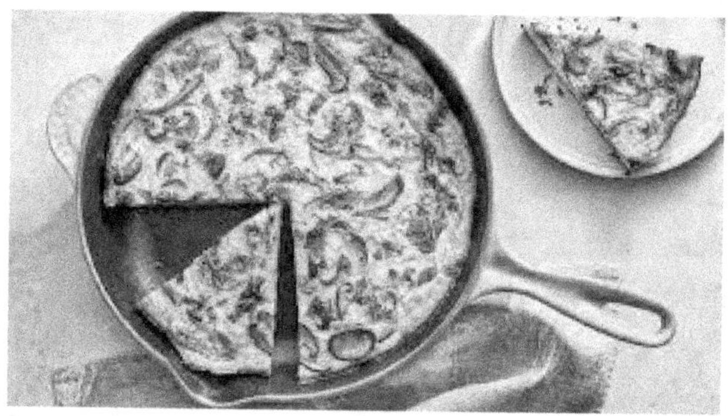

Ingredients:

- Six big eggs
- 1 cup fresh spinach leaves, chopped 1 cup mushrooms, sliced ½ onion, diced
- ¼ cup grated cheese (e.g., cheddar, feta, goat cheese)
- Two tablespoons of olive oil
- Salt & pepper, to taste
- Fresh herbs (e.g., parsley, chives) for garnish

Instructions:

1. **Preheat the Oven:**
   - Preheat your oven to 350°F (175°C).

2. **Sauté the Vegetables:**
   - Heat one tablespoon of olive oil over medium heat in an oven-safe skillet.
   - Add chopped onion and sliced mushrooms. Sauté until the mushrooms are soft and the onions are transparent approximately 3-4 minutes.

3. **Add Spinach:**
   - Add the chopped spinach to the skillet. Sauté for another 1-2 minutes until the spinach is wilted—season with a touch of salt and pepper.

4. **Whisk the Eggs:**
   - In a bowl, whisk the eggs until thoroughly blended—season with a touch of salt and pepper.

5. **Combine Eggs with Vegetables:**
   - Pour the whisked eggs over the sautéed veggies in the skillet. Gently toss to distribute the veggies properly.

6. **Add Cheese:**
   - Sprinkle the grated cheese over the egg and veggie mixture.
   - Cook on the Stovetop:

- Allow the frittata to cook on the stovetop for approximately 2 minutes or until the edges solidify.

7. **Transfer to Oven:**
   - Transfer the pan to the preheated oven and bake for 12-15 minutes, or until the frittata is firm in the middle and slightly browned on top.

8. **Garnish and Serve:**
   - Remove the frittata from the oven and let it cool for a few minutes.
   - Garnish with fresh herbs, if preferred.
   - Slice the frittata into wedges and serve warm.

9. **Enjoy:**
   - Your Spinach and Mushroom Frittata is ready to be enjoyed!

This frittata is a protein-packed breakfast option that contains healthful veggies. Spinach and mushrooms give vitamins, minerals, and antioxidants that help support your adrenal function and general wellness. Feel free to personalize the frittata with extra veggies, herbs, or spices to suit your preferences.

Nut Butter Banana Pancakes Recipe:

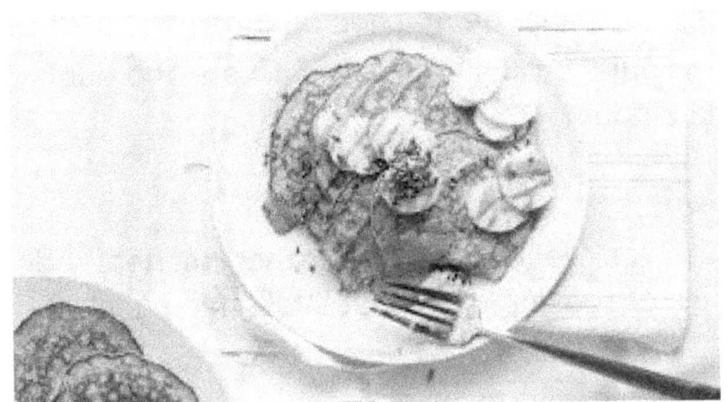

Ingredients:

- One ripe banana
- Two big eggs
- Two tablespoons nut butter (e.g., almond butter, peanut butter)
- ½ teaspoon vanilla extract
- ¼ teaspoon baking powder
- Pinch of salt
- Cooking oil (e.g., coconut oil) for cooking
- Toppings of your choosing (e.g., sliced bananas, berries, chopped almonds, maple syrup)

Instructions:

1. Mash the Banana:

- Mash the ripe banana with a fork until smooth in a mixing basin.

2. **Add Wet Ingredients:**
   - Add the eggs, nut butter, vanilla extract, baking powder, and a sprinkle of salt to the mashed banana.
   - Whisk the mixture until all components are thoroughly blended and smooth.

3. **Preheat the Pan:**
   - Heat a non-stick skillet or griddle over medium heat. Add a tiny quantity of cooking oil to coat the surface gently.

4. **Cook the Pancakes:**
   - Pour a bit of the batter onto the skillet to make a pancake. You may make the pancakes as big or tiny as you desire.
   - Cook for 2-3 minutes on one side until little bubbles appear on the surface.

5. **Flip and Cook:**
   - Carefully turn the pancake using a spatula and cook for another 1-2 minutes on the other side until golden brown and cooked through.

6. **Repeat:**
   - Repeat the cooking procedure with the remaining batter, adding extra oil to the pan as required.

7. **Serve and Top:**
   - Stack the Nut Butter Banana Pancakes on a platter.
   - Top with your favourite toppings, such as sliced bananas, berries, chopped nuts, and a drizzle of maple syrup.

- Your Nut Butter Banana Pancakes are ready to be enjoyed!

These pancakes combine protein from the eggs, healthy fats from the nut butter, and natural sweetness from the banana. This makes them a balanced and enjoyable breakfast that may support your adrenal health and deliver sustained energy throughout the morning. Customize the toppings to your taste for a beautiful and healthful start to your day.

Oat Bran Porridge Recipe:

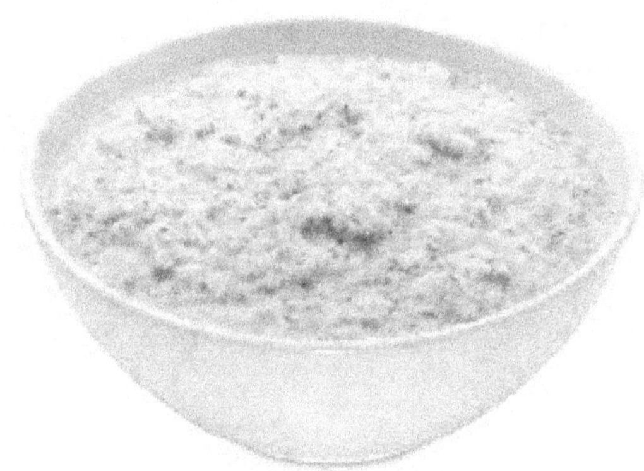

Ingredients:

- ½ cup oat bran
- 1 cup unsweetened almond milk (or any milk of your choice)
- ½ teaspoon vanilla extract
- Pinch of salt

- Toppings of your choice (e.g., sliced almonds, chopped apples, ground cinnamon, honey)

Instructions:

1. Combine Ingredients:
   - Mix oat bran, unsweetened almond milk, vanilla essence, and a bit of salt in a saucepan.

2. Cook the Porridge:
   - Place the pot over medium heat and bring the mixture to a moderate boil.
   - Stir periodically to avoid sticking. Cook for approximately 3-5 minutes or until the oat bran has thickened and achieved your preferred consistency.

3. Stir in Toppings:
   - Once the porridge is done, remove the pot from the heat.
   - Stir in your favourite toppings, such as sliced almonds, chopped apples, a sprinkle of ground cinnamon, and a drizzle of honey.

4. Serve:
   - Transfer the oat bran porridge to a bowl.
   - Add more toppings if desired.

5. Enjoy:
   - Your Oat Bran Porridge is ready to be enjoyed!

Oat bran is high in soluble fibre, which may help promote digestive health, control blood sugar levels, and create a sensation of fullness. Almonds, apples, and honey add to the porridge taste, nutrition, and sweetness. This warm and hearty meal may fuel your body and give you sustained energy for your day ahead. Feel free to modify the toppings depending on your tastes and dietary restrictions.

Veggie Breakfast Burrito Recipe:

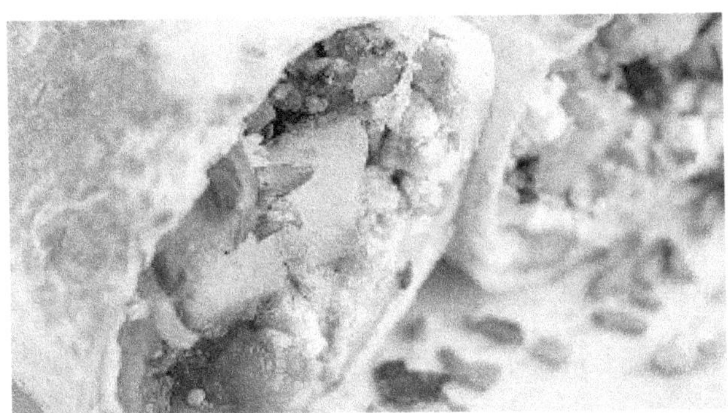

Ingredients:

- Two big whole-grain tortillas
- Four big eggs
- ½ cup sliced bell peppers (any colour)
- ½ cup chopped tomatoes
- ¼ cup chopped red onion
- ½ cup cooked black beans
- ½ cup shredded cheese (e.g., cheddar, pepper jack)
- One tablespoon of olive oil
- Salt & pepper, to taste

- Fresh cilantro for garnish (optional)
- Salsa or spicy sauce for serving (optional)

Instructions:

1. Sauté the Veggies:

   - In a pan, heat olive oil over medium heat.
   - Add chopped bell peppers, diced tomatoes, and diced red onion. Sauté for around 3-4 minutes, until the veggies are softened.

2. Scramble the Eggs:
   - Push the sautéed veggies to one side of the pan and break the eggs into the other.
   - Scramble the eggs with a spatula until they are cooked and combined with the veggies.

3. Add Black Beans:
   - Stir in the cooked black beans, letting them heat through.
   - Season and Assemble:

   - Season the mixture with salt and pepper to taste.

4. Warm Tortillas:
   - Warm the whole-grain tortillas quickly in a dry skillet or microwave.

5. **Assemble the Burritos:**
   - Divide the veggie and egg mixture between the tortillas, putting it in the middle of each.

6. **Add Cheese:**
   - Sprinkle shredded cheese over the veggie and egg mixture in each tortilla.

7. **Roll the Burritos:**
   - Fold in the edges of the tortillas and then wrap them up firmly to make burritos.

8. **Serve and Garnish:**
   - Place the Veggie Breakfast Burritos seam-side down on plates.
   - Garnish with fresh cilantro, if preferred.

9. **Serve with Salsa:**
   - Serve the burritos with salsa or spicy sauce on the side.

10. **Enjoy:**
   - Your Veggie Breakfast Burritos are ready to be enjoyed! This morning burrito is rich with protein from the eggs and black beans and fibre and minerals from the colourful veggies. It's a hearty and gratifying way to start your day with prolonged energy and adrenal support. Feel free to alter the ingredients and spices to meet your taste preferences.

Coconut Chia Pudding Recipe:

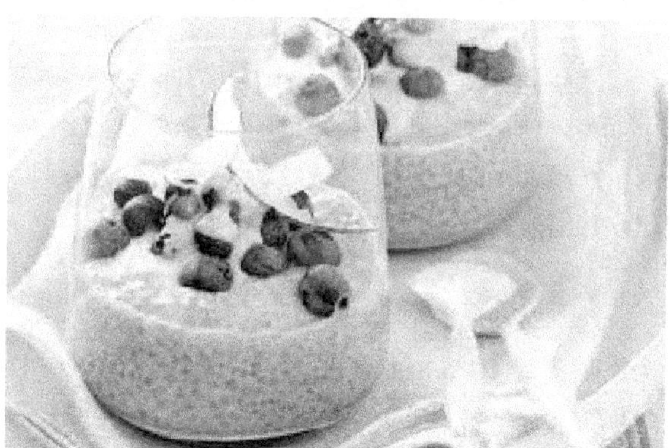

Ingredients:

- ¼ cup chia seeds
- 1 cup coconut milk (canned or carton)
- One tablespoon of honey or maple syrup (optional for sweetness)
- 1/2 teaspoon vanilla extract
- Fresh fruit (e.g., mango slices, berries) for topping
- Shredded coconut or chopped almonds for topping (optional)

Instructions:

1. Mix Chia Seeds and Liquid:
   - In a bowl, blend chia seeds, coconut milk, honey or maple syrup (if using), and vanilla essence.

2. **Stir and Let Sit:**
   - Stir the mixture carefully to distribute the chia seeds properly.
   - Let the mixture settle for approximately 5 minutes, then whisk again to avoid clumping.

3. **Refrigerate and Wait:**
   - Cover the bowl and refrigerate the mixture for at least 2 hours or overnight.
   - The chia seeds will absorb the liquid during this time and develop a pudding-like consistency.

4. **Serve and Top:**
   - When ready to serve, thoroughly toss the chia pudding to ensure it's properly blended.
   - Spoon the chia pudding into serving dishes or glasses.

5. **Add Fresh Fruit:**
   - Top the chia pudding with fresh fruit, such as mango slices or berries.

6. **Optional Toppings:**
   - Put shredded coconut or chopped almonds on top for extra texture and taste if desired.

7. **Enjoy:**
   - Your Coconut Chia Pudding is ready to be enjoyed!

Chia seeds are rich in fibre, omega-3 fatty acids, and antioxidants, making them a fantastic addition to your diet for adrenal health. The chia seeds and coconut milk mix give healthy fats and lasting energy to start your day. The fresh fruit topping provides natural sweetness and added vitamins. Feel free to tweak the sweetness and toppings to your taste preferences.

Almond Flour Waffles

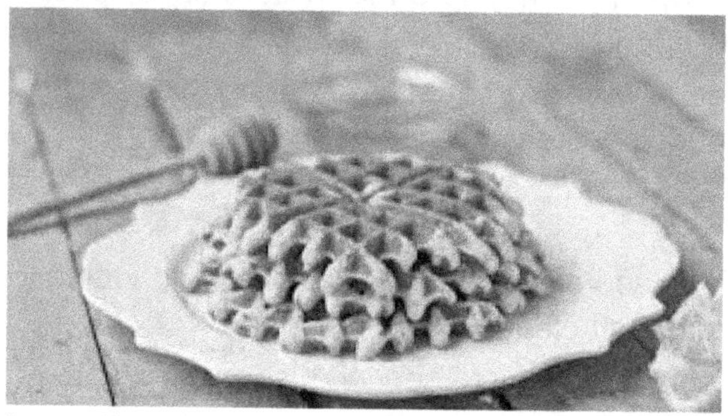

Ingredients:

- 1 cup almond flour
- ½ teaspoon baking powder
- Pinch of salt, two giant eggs
- ¼ cup unsweetened almond milk (or any milk of your choice)
- One tablespoon of melted coconut oil or butter
- One teaspoon of vanilla extract
- **Optional:** a touch of sweetness (e.g., honey, maple syrup)

Instructions:

1. **Preheat the Waffle Iron:**
    - Preheat your waffle iron according to the manufacturer's directions.

2. **Combine Dry Ingredients:**
    - Whisk together almond flour, baking powder, and a touch of salt in a mixing bowl.

3. **Add Wet Ingredients:**
    - Mix eggs, almond milk, melted coconut oil or butter, vanilla extract, and any optional sweetener you choose in a separate dish.

4. **Combine Wet with Dry:**
    - Gradually add the wet components to the dry ingredients, stirring until completely incorporated. The batter should be smooth and somewhat thick.

5. **Cook the Waffles:**
    - Lightly coat the waffle iron with cooking spray or a small quantity of coconut oil.
    - Pour a part of the batter into the middle of the waffle iron, following the manufacturer's directions for your waffle iron's size.

6. **Cook till Golden Brown:**

- Close the waffle iron and cook the waffle until it's golden brown and crunchy. The cooking time will vary depending on your waffle iron.

7. **Repeat with Remaining Batter:**

- Repeat the cooking procedure with the remaining batter, greasing the waffle iron as required.

8. **Serve:**

- Once all the waffles are cooked, move them to serving dishes.

9. **Toppings:**

- Add your favourite toppings, such as fresh berries, sliced bananas, a dollop of Greek yoghurt, or a drizzle of honey.

10. **Enjoy:**

- Your Almond Flour Waffles are ready to be enjoyed!

Almond flour adds a nutty taste and nutritional density to these waffles, giving them a terrific source of protein, healthy fats, and dietary fibre. The waffles may be personalized with your choice of toppings to suit your taste preferences and create a balanced and wholesome meal.

Sardine Avocado Toast Recipe:

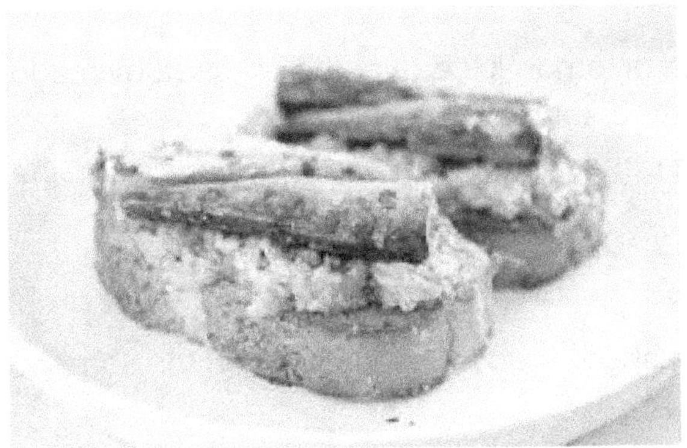

Ingredients:

- Two slices of whole-grain bread
- One ripe avocado
- One can of sardines (packed in water or olive oil), drained
  Lemon juice
- Salt & pepper, to taste
- **Optional toppings:** red onion slices, chopped parsley, chilli flakes

Instructions:

1. Toast the Bread:
    - Toast the pieces of whole-grain bread until they are crispy and golden brown.

2. Prepare the Avocado:
    - Cut the ripe avocado in halves, remove the pit, and scoop the flesh into a dish.

- Mash the avocado with a fork until smooth.

3. **Season the Avocado:**
    - Squeeze a dab of lemon juice over the mashed avocado to enhance taste and prevent browning.
    - Add a sprinkle of salt and pepper to taste, and combine thoroughly.

4. **Assemble the Toast:**
    - Spread the mashed avocado equally over the toasted bread pieces.

5. **Add Sardines:**
    - Place sardines on top of the avocado layer. You can split them into smaller pieces.

6. **Additional Toppings:**
    - Add sliced red onion, minced parsley, or a sprinkling of chilli flakes for added flavour and texture.

7. **Serve:**
    - Place the Sardine Avocado Toast on a platter.

8. **Enjoy:**
    - Your Sardine Avocado Toast is ready to be enjoyed!

This combo delivers a mix of healthful fats from the avocado and sardines, along with protein and omega-3 fatty acids from the sardines. Avocado also includes potassium and fibre, making it a healthy option for adrenal health. The whole-grain bread delivers complex carbs for lasting energy. Customize the toppings and spices to suit your taste preferences for a great and healthy breakfast.

Protein-Packed Breakfast Bowl Recipe

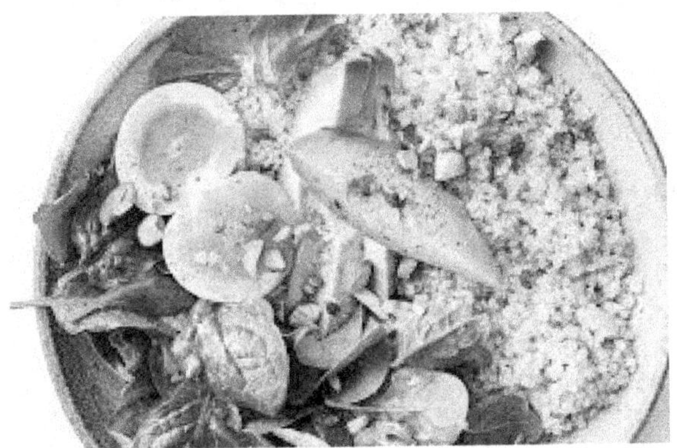

Ingredients:

- Cooked quinoa or brown rice
- Scrambled eggs (or tofu scramble for a vegan alternative)
- Sautéed spinach or kale
- Sliced avocado
- Diced tomatoes
- Black beans (canned or cooked)
- Crumbled feta cheese (optional)
- Pumpkin seeds or sunflower seeds
- Salt & pepper, to taste
- Olive oil or avocado oil for sautéing
- Optional toppings: spicy sauce, salsa, herbs

Instructions:

1. **Prepare the Components:**
   - Cook quinoa or brown rice according to package directions.
   - Prepare scrambled eggs or tofu scramble using your favourite technique.
   - Sauté spinach or kale in a touch of olive oil until wilted.

2. **Assemble the Bowl:**
   - Start by stacking a cooked quinoa or brown rice foundation in a dish.

3. **Add Protein:**
   - Top the oats with scrambled eggs or tofu scramble for a protein boost.

4. **Layer with Veggies:**
   - Add sautéed spinach or kale, sliced avocado, chopped tomatoes, and black beans to the bowl.

5. **Sprinkle with Seeds:**
   - Sprinkle pumpkin seeds or sunflower seeds on top for extra texture and nutrition.

6. **Add Cheese (Optional):**
   - If desired, grate feta cheese over the dish for added taste.

7. **Season and Garnish:**
   - Season the bowl with salt and pepper to taste.
   - Garnish with fresh herbs, if available.

8. **Optional Toppings:**
   - Drizzle with spicy sauce or salsa for added flavour and kick.

9. **Serve:**
   - Serve the Protein-Packed Breakfast Bowl immediately.

10. **Enjoy:**
    - Your Protein-Packed Breakfast Bowl is ready to be enjoyed!

This breakfast bowl contains nutritious carbs from quinoa or brown rice, protein from eggs or tofu, and various colourful veggies for vitamins and minerals. The beneficial fats from avocado and seeds and fibre from beans and vegetables make this bowl a balanced and pleasant option for adrenal health. Customize the ingredients and amounts depending on your tastes and dietary requirements.

CHAPTER FOUR

Sustaining Snacks

Chia Seed Pudding Parfait Recipe

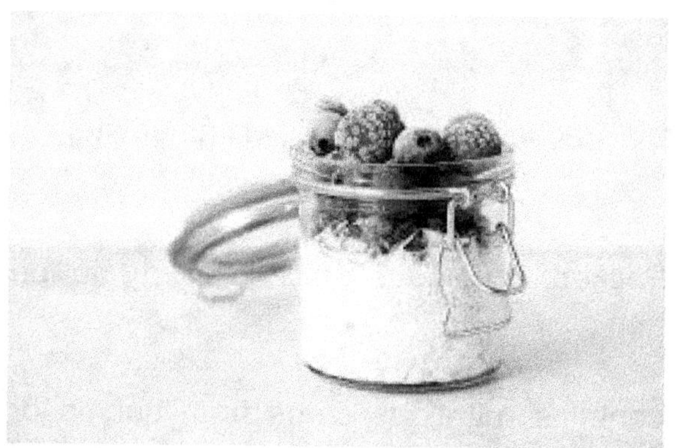

Ingredients:

For the Chia Seed Pudding:
- 3 tbsp chia seeds
- 1 cup unsweetened almond milk (or any milk of your choice)
- ½ teaspoon vanilla extract
- Optional: a bit of sweetness (e.g., honey, maple syrup)

For the Parfait Layers:
- Mixed berries (e.g., strawberries, blueberries, raspberries)
- Sliced banana

- Greek yoghurt or dairy-free yoghurt
- Nuts or seeds (e.g., almonds, walnuts, sunflower seeds)
- Granola (optional, for crunch)

Instructions:

1. **Prepare the Chia Seed Pudding:**
   - Blend chia seeds, almond milk, vanilla extract, and any optional sweetener in a dish.
   - Stir well to blend and make sure the chia seeds are appropriately distributed.
   - Let the mixture settle for approximately 5 minutes, then whisk again to avoid clumping.
   - Cover the bowl and refrigerate the mixture for at least 2 hours or overnight.

2. **Assemble the Parfait:**
   - Pick a glass or bowl for layering once the chia seed pudding has been set.
3. **Layer the Ingredients:**
   - Start by adding a scoop of chia seed pudding as the first layer.
   - Add a layer of mixed berries on top of the chia seed pudding.
   - Follow with a layer of sliced banana.

4. **Add Yogurt Layer:**
   - Spoon a layer of Greek or dairy-free yoghurt on the banana layer.

5. **Repeat Layers:**
   - Add another layer of chia seed pudding on top of the yoghurt layer.
   - Add another layer of mixed berries.

6. **Top with Nuts and Granola:**
   - Sprinkle a handful of chopped nuts or seeds on the fruit layer for extra crunch and nutrients.
   - If desired, add a coating of granola for added texture.

7. **Serve and Enjoy:**
   - Your Chia Seed Pudding Parfait is ready to be enjoyed as a pleasant and nutrient-rich snack.

This parfait delivers a mix of fibre, healthy fats, protein, and antioxidants from chia seeds, berries, almonds, and yoghurt. It's a flexible snack personalized with your favourite fruits, yoghurt varieties, and toppings. Feel free to change the amounts and ingredients to suit your taste preferences and nutritional demands.

Veggie Sticks with Guacamole Snack:

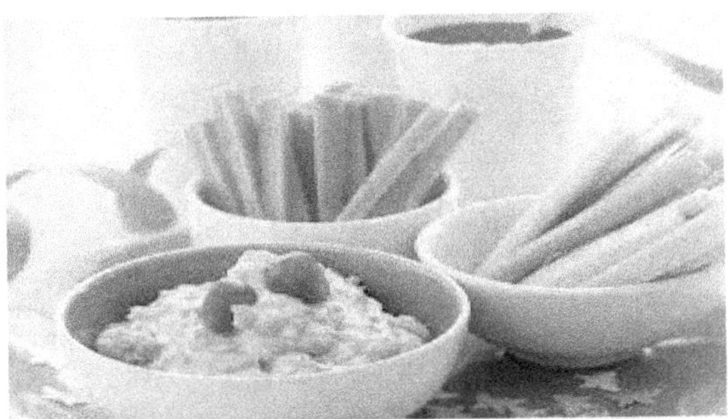

Ingredients:

1. For the Guacamole:
   - Two ripe avocados
   - One small tomato, chopped
   - ¼ red onion, coarsely chopped
   - One clove of garlic, minced Juice of 1 lime
   - Salt & pepper, to taste
   - Fresh cilantro, chopped (optional)

2. For the Veggie Sticks:
   - Carrot sticks
   - Cucumber sticks
   - Bell pepper sticks
   - Celery sticks

Instructions:

1. Prepare the Guacamole:
   - Cut the avocados in half, remove the pit, and scoop the flesh into a basin.
   - Mash the avocados with a fork until smooth.

2. Add Fresh Ingredients:
   - Add diced tomato, chopped red onion, minced garlic, and chopped cilantro (if using) to the mashed avocado.

3. Add Lime Juice and Season:
   - Squeeze the Juice of one lime over the mixture.
   - Season with salt and pepper to taste.

4. Mix Well:
   - Gently whisk all the ingredients together until thoroughly blended.

5. Prepare Veggie Sticks:
   - Wash and peel the veggies as required.
   - Cut carrot, cucumber, bell pepper, and celery into sticks.

6. Serve Guacamole with Veggie Sticks:
   - Place the guacamole in a bowl and arrange the vegetable sticks around it.

7. Dip and Enjoy:
   - Dip the vegetable sticks into the guacamole and enjoy this tasty, nutrient-rich snack.

Guacamole is rich in heart-healthy fats from avocados, while vegetable sticks add vitamins, minerals, and nutritional fibre. This combo delivers a mix of nutrients and tastes that may fulfil your appetites while boosting adrenal health. Customize the guacamole components to your preference, and feel free to experiment with different veggie selections as well.

Turkey or Chicken Wraps Snack:

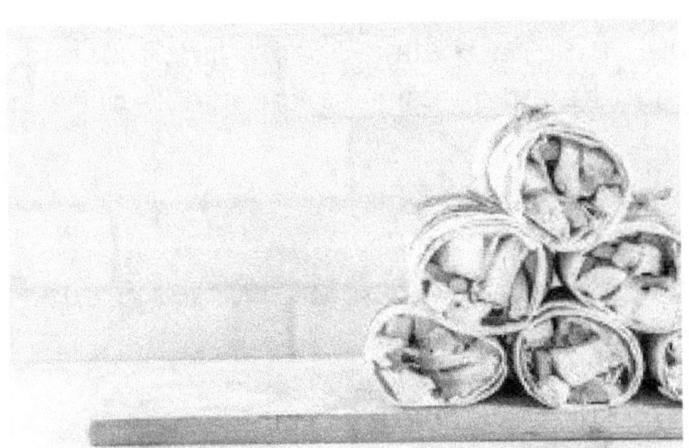

Ingredients:

For the Wraps:
   - Whole-grain tortillas or wraps
   - Sliced turkey breast or roasted chicken breast
   - Lettuce leaves (e.g., romaine, spinach)
   - Sliced tomato Sliced cucumber

- Optional: sliced avocado, red onion, cheese

For the Spread (optional):

-
- Hummus Mustard Greek yoghurt-based dressing

Instructions:

1. **Prepare the Ingredients:**
   - Lay out the whole-grain tortillas or wraps on a clean surface.

2. **Spread the Dressing (Optional):**
   - If preferred, apply a slight coating of hummus, mustard, or a Greek yoghurt-based dressing on the middle of each tortilla.

3. **Layer the Fillings:**
   - Lay the sliced turkey or chicken breast over the Spread, producing a uniform layer.

4. **Add Fresh Veggies:**
   - Place lettuce leaves, sliced tomato, and sliced cucumber on top of the protein.

5. **Optional Additions:**
   - Add sliced avocado, red onion, and a sprinkling of cheese for added taste and benefits if preferred.

6. **Fold and Roll:**
   - Fold in the edges of the tortilla, then roll it up firmly from the bottom, enclosing the ingredients.

7. **Cut and Serve:**
   - If desired, split the wrap in half diagonally for better handling.

8. **Enjoy:**
   - Your Turkey or Chicken Wrap is ready to be enjoyed as a pleasant and protein-rich snack.

Turkey or chicken wraps give a fantastic dose of lean protein, complete grains, and various colourful veggies. These portable wraps make them an excellent alternative for busy days when you need a fast and balanced snack to support your adrenal health. Customize the ingredients and condiments according to your tastes and dietary restrictions.

Rice Cake with Nut Butter and Berries Snack:

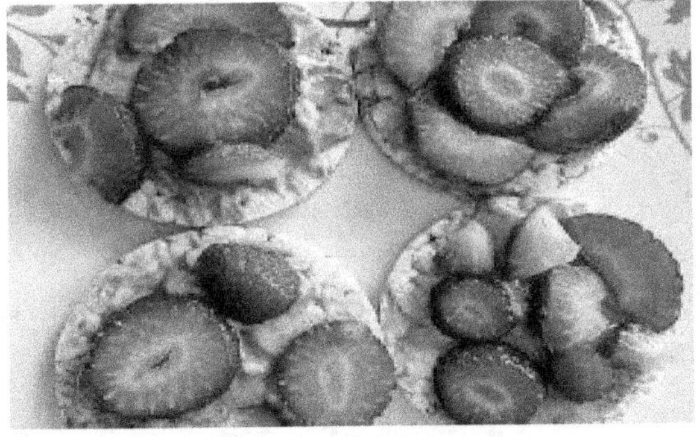

Ingredients:

- Rice cakes (simple or whole-grain)
- Nut butter (e.g., almond butter, peanut butter)
- Mixed berries (e.g., strawberries, blueberries, raspberries)
- **Optional:** drizzle of honey or sprinkle of cinnamon

Instructions:

1. Choose a Rice Cake:
   - Select plain or whole-grain rice cakes as your basis.

2. Spread Nut Butter:
   - Spread a layer of nut butter (such as almond or peanut butter) onto the rice cake.

3. Add Mixed Berries:
   - Arrange a selection of mixed berries on top of the nut butter layer.

4. Optional Sweetener or Spice:
   - If preferred, pour some honey over the berries for sweetness or sprinkle a dash of cinnamon for extra flavour.

5. Serve and Enjoy:
   - Your Rice Cake with Nut Butter and Berries is ready to be enjoyed as a nutritious and delightful snack.

This snack delivers a blend of complex carbs from the rice cake, healthy fats and protein from the nut butter, and vitamins and antioxidants from the mixed berries. It's a terrific option for people searching for a fast and balanced snack to support their adrenal health while enjoying a pleasant combination of tastes and textures. Feel free to alter the kind of nut butter and berries depending on your preferences and nutritional requirements.

Roasted Chickpea Salad:

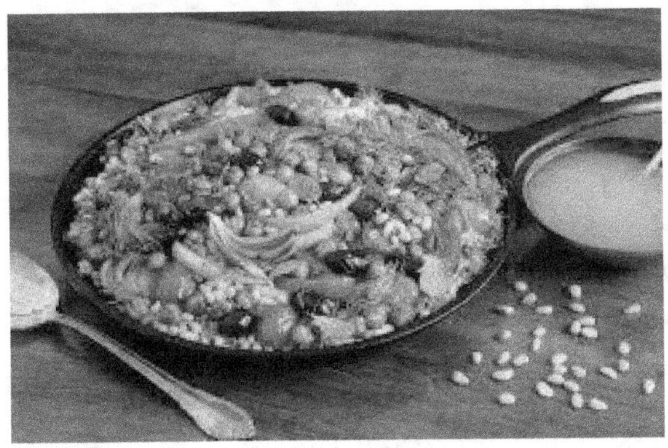

Ingredients:

For the Roasted Chickpeas:

- One can chickpeas (15 oz), drained and rinsed
- 1-2 tbsp olive oil
- One teaspoon of ground cumin
- ½ teaspoon smoked paprika
- Salt & pepper, to taste

For the Salad:

- Mixed salad greens (e.g., lettuce, spinach, arugula)
- Sliced cucumber
- Cherry tomatoes, halved
- Sliced bell peppers
- Red onion, thinly sliced Feta cheese, crumbled (optional)
- Lemon vinaigrette dressing (or dressing of your choice)

Instructions:

1. Prepare Roasted Chickpeas:

- Preheat the oven to 400°F (200°C).
- Pat the chickpeas dry with a paper towel.
- Combine chickpeas with olive oil, ground cumin, smoked paprika, salt, and pepper in a bowl.
- Spread the chickpeas on a baking sheet in a single layer.
- Roast in the oven for approximately 20-25 minutes or until crispy and golden.

2. Assemble the Salad:

- Add mixed salad greens, sliced cucumber, cherry tomatoes, sliced bell peppers, and red onion in a large salad bowl.

Add Roasted Chickpeas:

Once the roasted chickpeas are cooked, let them cool slightly.

Add the roasted chickpeas to the salad.

Optional Cheese Topping:

If using, add crumbled feta cheese over the salad.

Drizzle Dressing:

Drizzle lemon vinaigrette dressing or your chosen dressing over the salad.

3. **Toss and Serve:**
   - Toss the salad ingredients together to blend everything evenly.

4. **Serve and Enjoy:**
   - Your Roasted Chickpea Salad can be a crisp and tasty supper or snack.

This salad delivers a mix of fibre and plant-based protein from roasted chickpeas and a variety of bright veggies that supply vitamins and minerals. The salad may be modified to your taste preferences by adding your favourite veggies, nuts, seeds, or even a protein source. Enjoy this healthy and tasty choice to boost your adrenal health.

Cherry Tomatoes with Mozzarella Snack:

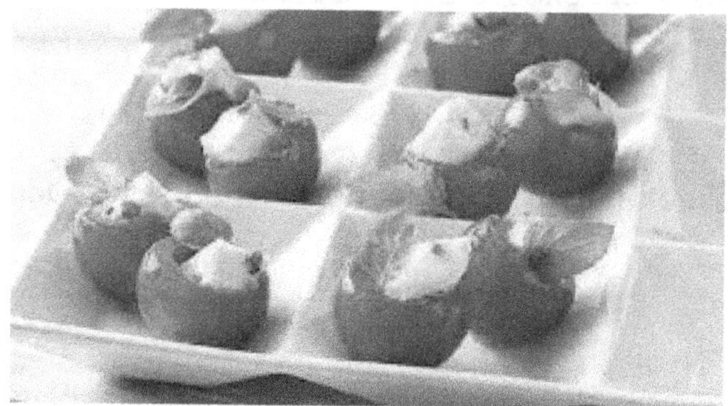

Ingredients:

- Cherry tomatoes
- Fresh mozzarella balls (bocconcini or little mozzarella pearls)
- Fresh basil leaves
- Balsamic vinegar or balsamic glaze
- Extra-virgin olive oil
- Salt & pepper, to taste

Instructions:

1. Prepare Cherry Tomatoes with Mozzarella:
   - Wash the cherry tomatoes and pat them dry.
   - Drain the fresh mozzarella balls if using bocconcini or little mozzarella pearls.

2. **Assemble the Skewers:**
   - If using skewers, thread a cherry tomato, a mozzarella ball, and a fresh basil leaf onto each skewer.
   - Alternatively, you may place the tomatoes and mozzarella on a dish.

3. **Drizzle with Dressing:**
   - Drizzle a balsamic vinegar or balsamic glaze over the cherry tomatoes and mozzarella.

4. **Add Olive Oil and Season:**
   - Drizzle a tiny quantity of extra-virgin olive oil over the snack.
   - Season with a bit of salt and pepper to taste.

5. **Garnish with Basil:**
   - Garnish the snack with more fresh basil leaves for added taste and colour.

6. **Serve and Enjoy:**
   - Your Cherry Tomatoes with Mozzarella snack is ready to be enjoyed as a refreshing and savoury alternative.

This snack delivers a blend of luscious cherry tomatoes, creamy mozzarella, and fragrant basil, all accentuated by the balsamic vinegar and olive oil. It's a light and delicious meal that delivers a mix of tastes and nutrients, making it appropriate for maintaining adrenal health. Feel free to change the quantity and seasoning according to your preferences.

Whole-Grain Crackers with Tuna Snack:

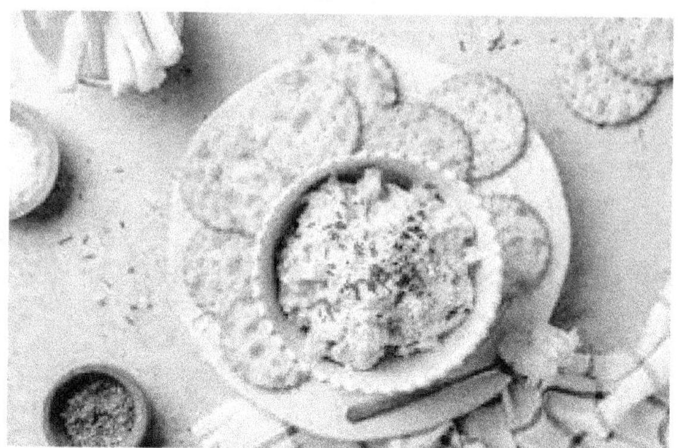

Ingredients:

- Whole-grain crackers
- Canned tuna (in water or olive oil), drained Lemon juice
- Diced red onion (optional)
- Chopped celery (optional)
- Dijon mustard (optional)
- Salt & pepper, to taste

Instructions:

1. Prepare the Tuna:
   - Open the can of tuna and drain the contents.

2. Season the Tuna:
   - In a bowl, flake the tuna using a fork.
   - Add a squeeze of fresh lemon juice to improve the taste.

3. **Add Optional Ingredients:**
   - Add sliced red onion and chopped celery to the tuna for extra crunch and flavour if preferred.

4. **Add a Touch of Mustard:**
   - Add a tiny quantity of Dijon mustard and stir thoroughly for added flavour.

5. **Season with Salt & Pepper:**
   - Season the tuna mixture with a sprinkle of salt and pepper to taste.

6. **Assemble the Snack:**
   - Lay out whole-grain crackers on a dish.

7. **Top with Tuna:**
   - Spoon the seasoned tuna mixture onto the crackers.

8. **Serve and Enjoy:**
   - Your Whole-Grain Crackers with Tuna snack can be enjoyed as a protein-packed and delicious alternative.

This snack delivers a balance of lean protein from the tuna, complex carbs from the whole-grain crackers, and extra nutrients from the optional veggies. It's a terrific option for people wanting a balanced and tasty snack to promote adrenal health. Customize the tuna combination by adding things you love, and feel free to experiment with other flavours.

Oatmeal Energy Bites Recipe:

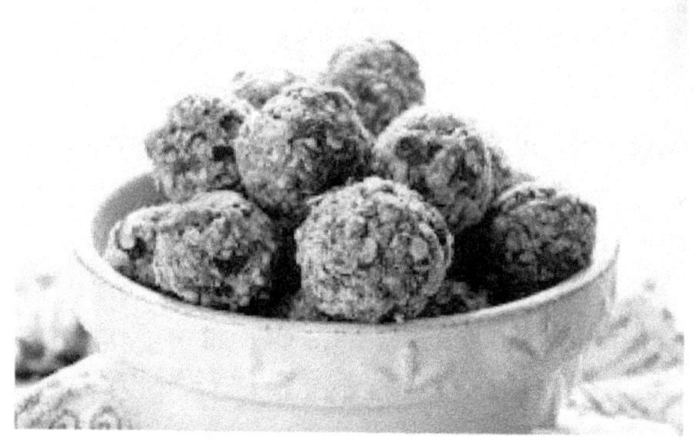

Ingredients:

- 1 cup rolled oats
- ½ cup nut butter (e.g., almond butter, peanut butter)
- 1/3 cup honey or maple syrup
- One teaspoon of vanilla extract
- ½ cup mix-ins (e.g., chopped nuts, dried fruits, chocolate chips, chia seeds)
- Pinch of salt (if using unsalted nut butter)

Instructions:

1. **Mix Wet Ingredients:**
   - Add nut butter, honey or maple syrup, and vanilla extract to a mixing dish.
   - If your nut butter is unsalted, add a touch of salt for taste.

2. **Add Rolled Oats:**
    - Stir in the rolled oats until thoroughly covered with the wet mixture.

3. **Add Mix-Ins:**
    - Add your choice of mix-ins, such as chopped nuts, dried fruits, chocolate chips, and chia seeds.
    - Mix everything until equally distributed.

4. **Chill the Mixture:**
    - Place the mixture in the refrigerator for approximately 30 minutes. This will make it easy to mould the energy bits.

5. **Shape the Energy Bites:**
    - Once the mixture has cold, use your hands to roll tiny parts of the dough into bite-sized balls.

6. **Store:**
    - Place the energy bits on a parchment-lined tray or dish.
    - You may eat them immediately or preserve them in an airtight jar in the refrigerator for up to a week.

7. **Enjoy:**
    - Your Oatmeal Energy Bites are ready to be enjoyed as a fast and healthy snack!

These energy bites are filled with whole-grain oats for continuous energy, nut butter for healthy fats and protein, and mix-ins for taste and texture. They're excellent for on-the-go munching or a fast pick-me-up. Customize the mix-ins to your taste preferences and nutritional restrictions for a unique snack experience.

Mixed Berries with Nuts Snack:

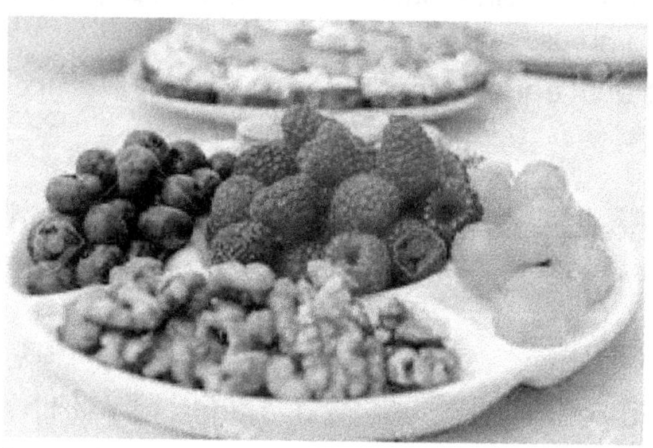

Ingredients:

- Mixed berries (e.g., strawberries, blueberries, raspberries, blackberries)
- Assorted nuts (e.g., almonds, walnuts, cashews, pistachios)
- **Optional:** a drizzle of honey or a sprinkling of cinnamon

Instructions:

1. Wash and Prepare Berries:
   - Wash the mixed berries under cold water and blot them dry with a paper towel.
   - If required, remove any stems or hulls from the berries.

2. Choose Nuts:

   - Select a selection of nuts or seeds to complement the berries. You may use one variety of nuts or make a combination.

3. Combine Berries with Nuts:

   - Place the mixed berries in a basin or on a platter.
   - Add a handful of mixed nuts on the side or spread them over the berries.

4. Optional Additions:

   - If desired, sprinkle a tiny quantity of honey over the berries for natural sweetness.
   - Alternatively, sprinkle a pinch of cinnamon over the mixture for extra taste.

5. Serve and Enjoy:

   - Your Mixed Berries with Nuts snack is ready to be enjoyed as a nutritious and pleasant alternative.

This snack delivers a blend of fresh, juicy berries rich in antioxidants and vitamins, combined with the beneficial fats, protein, and crunch from the nuts. It's a terrific way to enjoy a blast of natural sweetness and brilliant colours while boosting adrenal health. Customize the varieties of berries and nuts according to your tastes and nutritional requirements, and feel free to alter the serving amounts to suit your hunger.

Avocado Rice Cakes Snack:

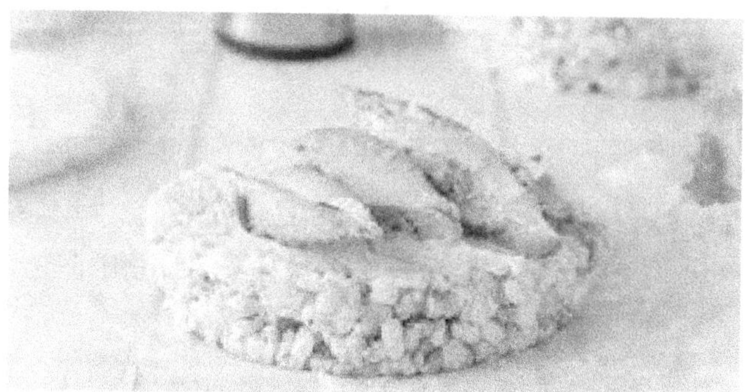

Ingredients:

- Rice cakes (simple or whole-grain)
- Ripe avocado
- Lemon juice
- Salt & pepper, to taste
- Optional toppings: red pepper flakes, microgreens, sliced radishes

Instructions:

1. Prepare Avocado:
   - Cut the ripe avocado in halves, remove the pit, and scoop the flesh into a dish.

2. Mash Avocado:
   - Mash the avocado with a fork until you obtain your desired consistency. Leave it somewhat lumpy, or make it smooth.

3. Season Avocado:
   - Squeeze a dab of lemon juice over the mashed avocado to enhance the taste and avoid browning.
   - Add a sprinkle of salt, salt, and pepper to taste, and combine thoroughly.

4. Assemble the Rice Cakes:
   - Lay out the rice cakes on a clean surface.

5. Spread Avocado:
   - Spread a liberal amount of mashed avocado onto each rice cake.

6. Optional Toppings:
   - Add a pinch of red pepper flakes for flavour and colour if desired.
   - Add microgreens or sliced radishes for added freshness and crunch.

7. Serve and Enjoy:
   - Your Avocado Rice Cakes are ready to be enjoyed as a simple and delightful snack.

This snack delivers the beneficial fats and creamy smoothness of avocado mixed with the crunch of rice cakes. It's a terrific choice for individuals searching for a balanced snack that delivers fullness and taste while boosting adrenal health. Customize the toppings and spices according to your preferences and dietary restrictions.

CHAPTER FIVE

Wholesome Lunches

Roasted Vegetable Quinoa Bowl:

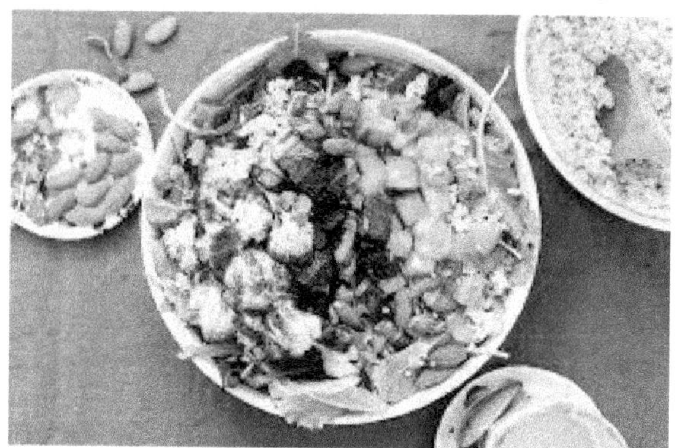

Ingredients:

For the Roasted Vegetables:
- Assorted veggies (e.g., bell peppers, zucchini, cherry tomatoes, broccoli)
- Olive oil
- Salt and pepper
- Optional: dried herbs (such as thyme, rosemary, or oregano)

For the Quinoa:

Cooked quinoa For the Dressing:
- Olive oil

- Lemon juice
- Dijon mustard
- Garlic, minced
- Salt and pepper

For Toppings (Optional):
- Crumbled feta cheese
- Toasted nuts or seeds (e.g., almonds, pumpkin seeds)
- Fresh herbs (e.g., parsley, basil)

Instructions:

1. Prepare the Vegetables:
   - Preheat the oven to 400°F (200°C).
   - Cut the different veggies into bite-sized pieces.
   - Toss the veggies with olive oil, salt, pepper, and dry herbs.
   - Spread the veggies on a baking sheet in a single layer.
   - Roast in the oven for approximately 20-25 minutes or until soft and slightly browned.

2. Make the Dressing:
   - Mix olive oil, lemon juice, Dijon mustard, minced Garlic, salt, and pepper in a separate bowl to make the dressing.

3. Assemble the Bowl:
   - In serving bowls, stack cooked quinoa as the basis.

4. Add Roasted Vegetables:
   - Top the quinoa with the roasted veggies.

5. **Drizzle with Dressing:**
   - Drizzle the dressing over the veggies and quinoa.

6. **Optional Toppings:**
   - Add crumbled feta cheese, roasted nuts or seeds, and fresh herbs over the dish if preferred.

7. **Serve and Enjoy:**
   - Your Roasted Vegetable Quinoa Bowl is ready to be enjoyed as a nutritious and enjoyable meal.

This bowl delivers a blend of fibre-rich quinoa, roasted veggies packed with antioxidants, and healthy fats from the dressing and optional toppings. It's a flexible alternative you can modify by combining your favourite veggies, seasonings, and extra protein sources like grilled chicken or chickpeas.

Tuna Salad Lettuce Wraps:

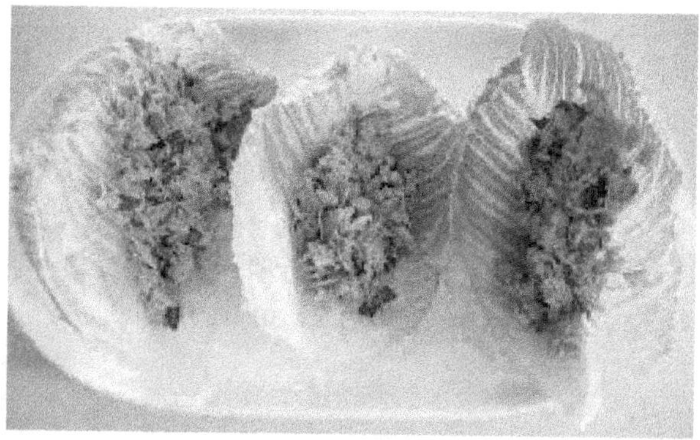

Ingredients:

For the Tuna Salad:
- Canned tuna (in water or olive oil), drained Greek yoghurt or mayonnaise (for smoothness)
- Chopped celery
- Chopped red onion
- Dill or parsley, chopped (optional)
- Lemon juice
- Salt & pepper, to taste

For Assembly:
- Large lettuce leaves (such as iceberg, romaine, or butter lettuce)
- Sliced Cucumber
- Sliced tomato

Instructions:

1. Prepare Tuna Salad:
   - Mix the drained canned tuna with Greek yoghurt or mayonnaise in a bowl.
   - Add chopped celery, diced red onion, chopped dill or parsley (if using), and a squeeze of lemon juice.
   - Season with salt, salt, and pepper to taste.
   - Mix everything until thoroughly blended.

2. Assemble the Lettuce Wraps:
   - Take a big lettuce leaf and arrange it flat on a clean table.

3. **Add Tuna Salad:**
    - Spoon a spoonful of the tuna salad into the middle of the lettuce leaf.

4. **Add Cucumber and Tomato:**
    - Add sliced Cucumber and sliced tomato on top of the tuna salad.

5. **Wrap and Secure:**
    - Fold in the sides of the lettuce leaf and then roll it up, producing a wrap.

6. **Serve and Enjoy:**
    - Your Tuna Salad Lettuce Wrap is ready to be enjoyed as a fresh and delightful meal.

These wraps provide a balanced blend of protein from the tuna, fibre from the veggies, and a crisp crunch from the lettuce. They're a terrific alternative for individuals wanting a lighter lunch that promotes adrenal health while offering necessary nutrients. Customize the ingredients and spices depending on your taste preferences and nutritional requirements.

Brown Rice Sushi Rolls (California Rolls)

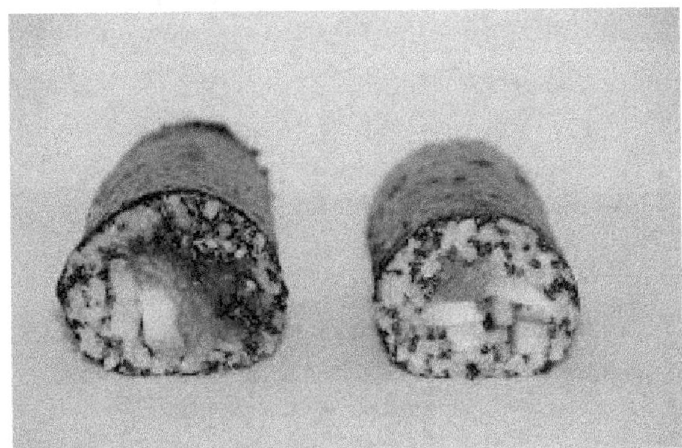

Ingredients:

For the Sushi Rice:

- Brown sushi rice
- Rice vinegar
- Sugar
- Salt

For Assembly:

- Nori seaweed sheets
- Cooked and seasoned brown sushi rice
- Imitation crab or genuine crab meat shredded
- Sliced avocado
- Cucumber, julienned
- **Optional:** roasted sesame seeds

For Dipping:

- Low-sodium soy sauce

- Wasabi and pickled Ginger (optional)

Instructions:

1. Prepare Sushi Rice:
   - Cook brown sushi rice according to the package directions.
   - In a bowl, combine rice vinegar, sugar, and salt salt.
   - Once the rice is cooked and has cooled, carefully whisk in the vinegar mixture to season the rice.

2. Assemble Sushi Rolls:
   - Lay a bamboo sushi rolling mat on a clean surface.
   - Place a sheet of nori seaweed on the mat, shiny side down.

3. Spread Rice on Nori:
   - Wet your hands to prevent the rice from sticking, and then spread a thin layer of brown sushi rice evenly over the nori, leaving approximately an inch of nori exposed at the top.

4. Add Fillings:
   - Place shredded imitation crab or crab meat, sliced avocado, and julienned Cucumber horizontally on the rice.

5. **Roll the Sushi:**
   - Start rolling the sushi from the bottom, using the bamboo mat to help you move securely.
   - As you approach the exposed strip of nori at the top, moisten it gently with water to help seal the roll.

6. **Slice the Rolls:**
   - Once the roll is snugly wrapped, slice it into bite-sized pieces with a sharp knife.

7. **Serve and Enjoy:**
   - Arrange the sushi rolls on a dish, sprinkle with toasted sesame seeds (if preferred), and serve with low-sodium soy sauce, wasabi, and pickled Ginger.

Brown Rice Sushi Rolls provide a blend of entire grains from brown rice, healthy fats from avocado, and protein from crab. These rolls are a unique and pleasurable way to ingest nutrient-rich foods while boosting adrenal health. Experiment with various fillings and dipping sauces to create your favourite sushi combinations.

Mixed Greens and Grilled Chicken Salad:

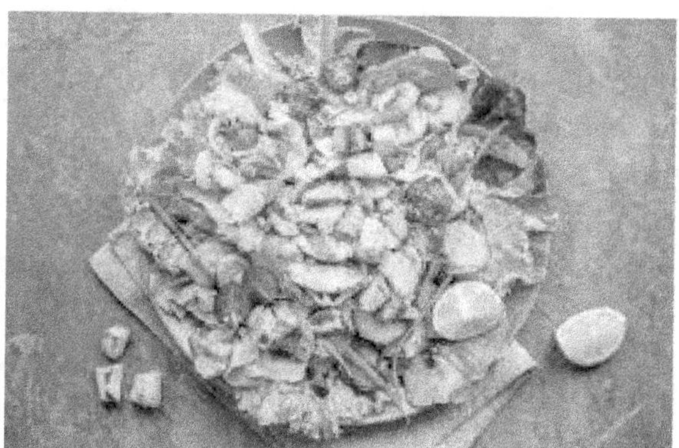

Ingredients:

For the Grilled Chicken:

- Boneless, skinless chicken breasts
- Olive oil, Lemon juice
- Garlic, minced
- Dried herbs (such as oregano, thyme, or rosemary)
- Salt and pepper

For the Salad:

- Mixed greens (e.g., lettuce, spinach, arugula)
- Sliced cherry tomatoes
- Sliced Cucumber
- Sliced bell peppers
- Red onion, thinly sliced
- **Optional add-ins:** almonds, seeds, avocado, feta cheese

For the Dressing:

- Olive oil
- Balsamic vinegar
- Dijon mustard
- Honey or maple syrup
- Salt and pepper

Instructions:

1. **Prepare Grilled Chicken:**
   - Preheat the grill or grill pan over medium-high heat.
   - Mix olive oil, lemon juice, minced Garlic, dried herbs, salt, salt, and pepper in a bowl.
   - Coat the chicken breasts with the marinade and let them marinate for 15-30 minutes.
   - Grill the chicken until cooked, approximately 6-8 minutes each side. Let it sit before slicing.

2. **Make the Dressing:**
   - Mix olive oil, balsamic vinegar, Dijon mustard, honey or maple syrup, salt, and pepper in a small bowl to make the dressing.

3. **Assemble the Salad:**
   - In a large salad bowl, put a bed of mixed greens.

4. **Add Vegetables and Toppings:**
   - Scatter sliced cherry tomatoes, sliced Cucumber, bell peppers, and red onion over the greens.

- Add nuts, seeds, avocado, and feta cheese for added taste and texture if preferred.

5. **Slice Grilled Chicken:**
   - Slice the grilled chicken breasts into thin pieces.

6. **Top with Chicken:**
   - Place the sliced grilled chicken on top of the salad.

7. **Drizzle with Dressing:**
   - Drizzle the balsamic dressing over the salad.

8. **Serve and Enjoy:**
   - Your Mixed Greens and Grilled Chicken Salad is ready to be enjoyed as a delightful and healthy meal.

This salad includes lush greens, colourful veggies, lean protein from grilled chicken, and healthy fats from optional toppings. The balsamic dressing gives a burst of flavour without sacrificing health advantages. Customize the salad with your chosen veggies and toppings to make a meal that meets your taste preferences and nutritional demands.

Black Bean and Sweet Potato Burrito Bowl:

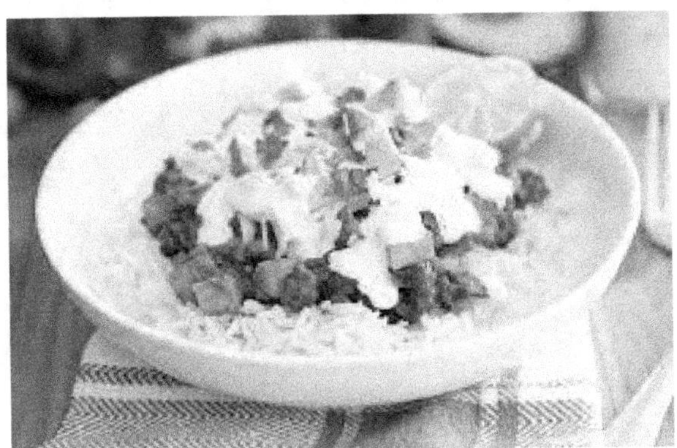

Ingredients:

For the Sweet Potatoes:

- Sweet potatoes, peeled and diced Olive oil
- Ground cumin
- Paprika
- Salt and pepper

For the Black Beans:

- Canned black beans, drained and rinsed Olive oil
- Garlic, minced
- Ground cumin
- Chili powder
- Salt and pepper

For the Assembly:

- Cooked brown rice or quinoa

- Sliced avocado
- Sliced bell peppers (assorted hues)
- Corn kernels (fresh, frozen, or canned)
- Sliced red onion
- Fresh cilantro leaves

For the Dressing:
- Lime juice
- Olive oil
- Ground cumin
- Salt and pepper

Instructions:

1. **Prepare Sweet Potatoes:**
   - Preheat the oven to 400°F (200°C).
   - Toss diced sweet potatoes with olive oil, ground cumin, paprika, salt, salt, and pepper.
   - Spread the sweet potatoes on a baking sheet and roast for approximately 20-25 minutes until soft and slightly crunchy.

2. **Prepare Black Beans:**
   - In a pan, heat olive oil over medium heat.
   - Add minced Garlic, ground cumin, chilli powder, salt, salt, and pepper. Cook for approximately 1 minute until aromatic.
   - Add drained black beans and simmer for a few minutes until cooked through.

3. **Make the Dressing:**
   - Mix lime juice, olive oil, ground cumin, salt, salt, and pepper in a separate bowl to make the dressing.

4. **Assemble the Bowl:**
   - Put cooked brown rice or quinoa as the basis in individual serving bowls.

5. **Add Sweet Potatoes and Black Beans:**
   - Top the grains with roasted sweet potatoes and sautéed black beans.

6. **Add Toppings:**
   - Add sliced avocado, bell peppers, corn kernels, and red onion to the bowl.

7. **Drizzle with Dressing:**
   - Drizzle the lime-cumin dressing over the bowl.

8. **Garnish and Serve:**
   - Garnish the dish with fresh cilantro leaves.

9. **Serve and Enjoy:**
   - Your Black Bean and Sweet Potato Burrito Bowl is ready to be enjoyed as a healthful and delightful meal.

This burrito bowl includes a blend of fibre-rich black beans, nutrient-packed sweet potatoes, and a variety of colourful veggies. The lime-cumin dressing adds a zesty flavour to the dish. Customize the toppings and spices depending on your tastes for a customized and fulfilling dinner that supports your adrenal health.

Egg Salad Stuffed Tomatoes:

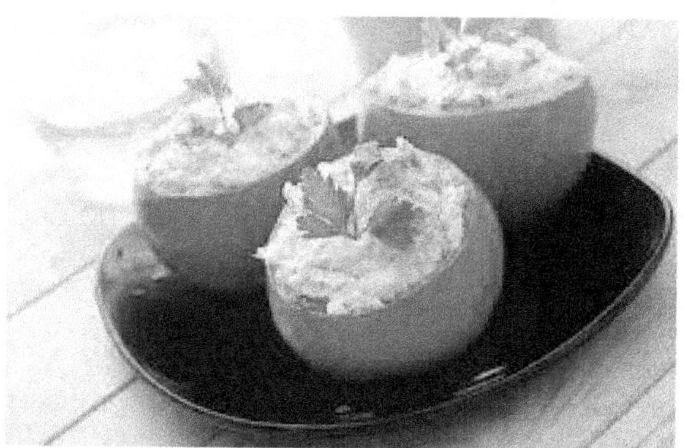

Ingredients:

For the Egg Salad:
- Hard-boiled eggs, peeled and chopped Greek yoghurt or mayonnaise (for smoothness)
- Dijon mustard
- Chopped fresh chives or green onions
- Salt & pepper, to taste

For the Tomatoes:
- Large ripe tomatoes

Salt and pepper, to taste For Garnish:
- Fresh herbs (such as parsley or dill)

- Paprika or smoked paprika (optional)

Instructions:

1. **Prepare Egg Salad:**
   - Add the chopped hard-boiled eggs, Greek yoghurt or mayonnaise, Dijon mustard, chopped chives or green onions, salt, salt, and pepper in a bowl.
   - Mix everything until thoroughly blended.

2. **Prepare Tomatoes:**
   - Cut the tops off the tomatoes and carefully scrape out the seeds and pulp, leaving a hollow hole for the egg salad.

3. **Season Tomatoes:**
   - Sprinkle the interior of the tomato shells with a touch of SaltSalt and pepper.

4. **Fill with Egg Salad:**
   - Spoon the egg salad mixture into the hollowed-out tomatoes.

5. **Garnish:**
   - Garnish the filled tomatoes with fresh herbs (such as parsley or dill) and a sprinkling of paprika or smoked paprika for extra taste and colour.

6. **Serve and Enjoy:**
   - Your Egg Salad Stuffed Tomatoes are ready to be enjoyed as a light and delightful meal.

These filled tomatoes give a protein-rich egg salad with creamy Greek yoghurt or mayonnaise paired with the refreshing juiciness of ripe tomatoes. They're a terrific alternative for a fast, tasty lunch promoting adrenal health. Customize the egg salad ingredients and spices to meet your tastes and dietary restrictions.

Chickpea and Vegetable Stir-Fry:

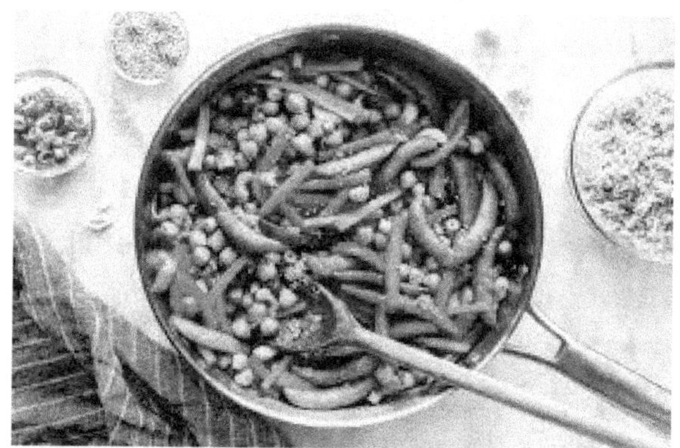

Ingredients:

1. For the Stir-Fry Sauce:
    - Low-sodium soy sauce
    - Sesame oil
    - Rice vinegar
    - Honey or maple syrup
    - Cornstarch (to thicken)
    - Crushed red pepper flakes (optional)

2. For the Stir-Fry:
   - Prepared chickpeas (canned or prepared from dry)
   - Assorted veggies (e.g., bell peppers, broccoli, snap peas, carrots), chopped Garlic, minced Ginger, minced Olive oil or cooking oil of choice
   - Cooked brown rice or quinoa

3. For Garnish (Optional):
   - Chopped green onions
   - Sesame seeds Instructions:

4. Prepare Stir-Fry Sauce:
   - Mix low-sodium soy sauce, sesame oil, rice vinegar, honey or maple syrup, cornstarch, and crushed red pepper flakes (if using). Set aside.

5. Stir-Fry the Vegetables:
   - Heat a large skillet or wok over medium-high heat.
   - Add a drizzle of olive oil or cooking oil to the skillet.
   - Add minced Garlic and minced Ginger, and sauté for approximately 30 seconds until aromatic.

6. Add Vegetables and Chickpeas:
   - Add the chopped veggies to the pan and stir-fry for a few minutes until they soften.
   - Add the cooked chickpeas and continue stir-frying until the veggies are tender-crisp.

7. Add Stir-Fry Sauce:
    - Pour the prepared stir-fry sauce over the veggies and chickpeas.
    - Stir thoroughly to coat the ingredients with the sauce.
    - Allow the sauce to thicken somewhat.

8. Serve with Grains:
    - Serve the chickpea and vegetable stir-fry over cooked brown rice or quinoa.

9. Garnish and Enjoy:
    - Garnish the stir-fry with chopped green onions and sesame seeds for extra taste and aesthetic appeal.

10. Serve and Enjoy:
    - Your Chickpea and Vegetable Stir-Fry is ready to be enjoyed as a delightful and healthy meal.

This stir-fry delivers a mix of plant-based protein from chickpeas, a range of bright veggies rich in vitamins and minerals, and a flavorful stir-fry sauce. It's a flexible recipe you can create by combining your favourite veggies and altering the amount of spice. Enjoy it as a pleasant and adrenal health-supportive dinner.

Greek Salad with Grilled Halloumi

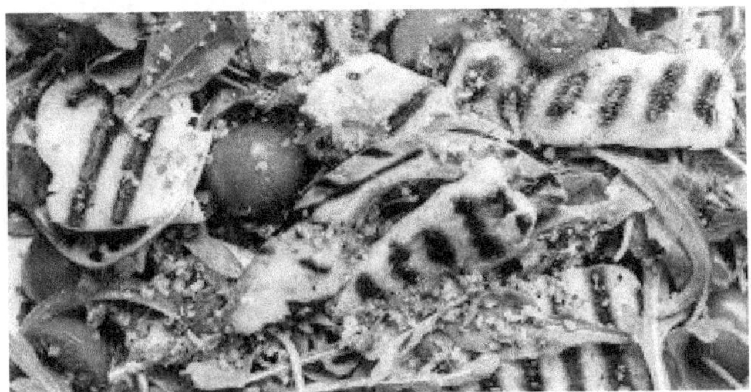

Ingredients:

1. For the Grilled Halloumi:
    * Halloumi cheese sliced Olive oil
    * Lemon juice
    * Dried oregano
    * Pepper

2. For the Greek Salad:
    * Mixed greens (e.g., lettuce, spinach, arugula),
    * Cherry tomatoes, halved Cucumber, diced Red onion, thinly sliced Kalamata olives, pitted Feta cheese, crumbled.

3. Fresh parsley or dill, chopped For the Dressing:
    * Olive oil
    * Red wine vinegar
    * Dried oregano

- Salt and pepper
- Instructions:

4. **Prepare Grilled Halloumi:**
   - Preheat a grill or grill pan over medium-high heat.
   - Mix olive oil, lemon juice, dried oregano, and a bit of pepper in a bowl.
   - Brush the halloumi slices with the olive oil mixture.
   - Grill the halloumi on each side for approximately 1-2 minutes until grill marks develop and the cheese is slightly melted.

5. **Prepare Greek Salad:**
   - In a large salad bowl, put a bed of mixed greens.

6. **Add Vegetables and Toppings:**
   - Scatter halved cherry tomatoes, diced Cucumber, thinly sliced red onion, Kalamata olives, crumbled feta cheese, and chopped fresh parsley or dill over the greens.

7. **Make the Dressing:**
   - Mix olive oil, red wine vinegar, dried oregano, salt, salt, and pepper in a small bowl to make the dressing.

8. **Drizzle with Dressing:**
   - Drizzle the dressing over the salad.

9. **Add Grilled Halloumi:**
   - Arrange the grilled halloumi slices on top of the salad.

10. Serve and Enjoy:

- Your Greek Salad with Grilled Halloumi is ready to be enjoyed as a delightful and savoury meal.

This salad delivers a beautiful combination of textures and tastes, with the creamy and slightly salty grilled halloumi complimenting the colourful veggies and acidic dressing. It's an excellent alternative for people wishing to have a Mediterranean-inspired supper that promotes adrenal health. Customize the salad ingredients depending on your tastes and dietary requirements.

Zucchini Noodles with Pesto and Chicken:

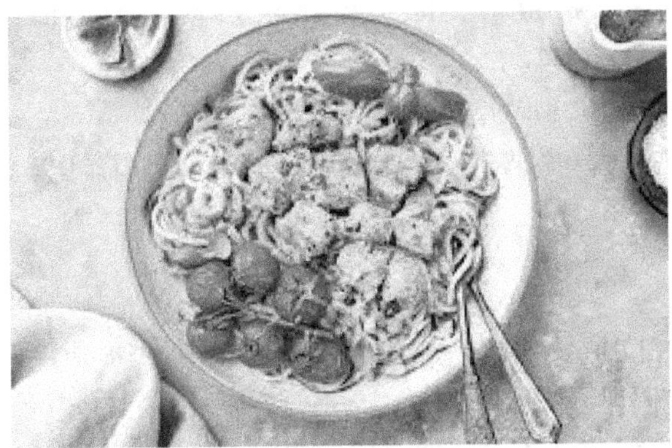

Ingredients:

For the Pesto:

- Fresh basil leaves
- Pine nuts or walnuts

- Garlic, minced Parmesan cheese, grated Olive oil
- Lemon juice
- Salt and pepper

For the Zucchini Noodles:
- Zucchini spiralized into noodles
- Cooked chicken breast, cut or diced Cherry tomatoes, halved Olive oil
- Salt and pepper

Instructions:

1. Prepare Pesto:
   - In a food processor, blend fresh basil leaves, pine nuts or walnuts, chopped Garlic, grated Parmesan cheese, and a drizzle of olive oil.
   - Pulse the ingredients until they create a coarse paste.
   - Add lemon juice, salt, and pepper to taste, and pulse again to blend.

2. Prepare Zucchini Noodles:
   - Spiralize the zucchini into noodle-like strands using a spiralizer or julienne peeler.
   - Heat a skillet over medium heat and add a drizzle of olive oil.
   - Add the zucchini noodles and sauté for a few minutes until they are barely soft. Be cautious not to overcook.

3. **Combine with Chicken and Tomatoes:**
   - Add the cooked chicken breast pieces or diced chicken to the pan with the zucchini noodles.
   - Toss the halved cherry tomatoes and gently cook until the chicken is warmed.

4. **Add Pesto:**
   - Stir in the prepared pesto sauce, completely covering the noodles and chicken.

5. **Serve and Enjoy:**
   - Your Zucchini Noodles with Pesto and Chicken are ready to be enjoyed as a light and savoury lunch.

This meal gives a new spin on conventional pasta by combining zucchini noodles and a handmade pesto sauce. It's a terrific way to add veggies to your supper while enjoying the pleasant taste of pesto and grilled chicken. Customize the recipe using your preferred protein and tweak the pesto components to meet your taste preferences.

CHAPTER SIX

Nourishing Dinners

Grilled Salmon with Quinoa and Roasted Vegetables:

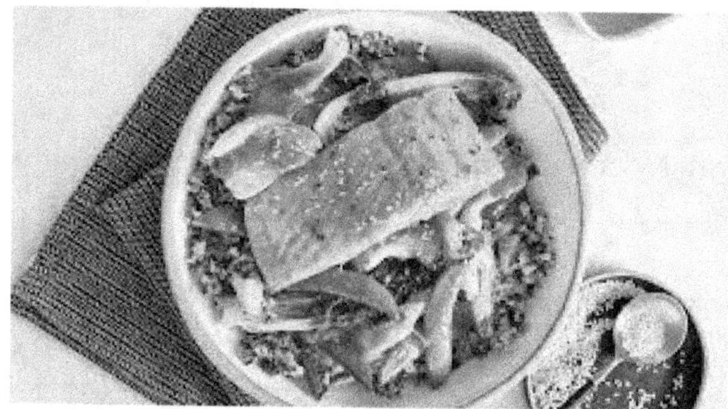

Ingredients:

For the Grilled Salmon:
- Salmon fillets
- Olive oil
- Lemon juice
- Fresh herbs (such as dill, parsley, or thyme)
- Salt and pepper

For the Quinoa:
- Quinoa Vegetable broth or water Salt.

For the Roasted Vegetables:

- Assorted veggies (e.g., bell peppers, zucchini, carrots, broccoli)
- Olive oil
- Dried herbs (such as rosemary or thyme)
- Salt and pepper

Instructions:

1. **Prepare Quinoa:**
   - Rinse the quinoa well in cold water.
   - In a saucepan, blend quinoa and vegetable broth (or water) in a 2:1 ratio (2 parts liquid to 1 part quinoa).
   - Add a pinch of salt and bring to a boil. Reduce heat, cover, and simmer for approximately 15-20 minutes, or until the quinoa is cooked and the liquid is absorbed.

2. **Prepare Grilled Salmon:**
   - Preheat the grill to medium-high heat.
   - Combine olive oil, lemon juice, chopped fresh herbs, salt, salt, and pepper in a bowl.
   - Brush the salmon fillets with the olive oil mixture.
   - Grill the salmon for approximately 4-6 minutes on each side or until cooked to your optimum amount of doneness.

3. **Roast Vegetables:**
   - Preheat the oven to 400°F (200°C).
   - Chop the varied veggies into bite-sized pieces.

- Toss the veggies with olive oil, dried herbs, salt, salt, and pepper.
- Spread the veggies on a baking sheet in a single layer and roast for approximately 20-25 minutes or until soft and slightly browned.

4. **Assemble the Dish:**
   - In individual serving dishes, make a bed of cooked quinoa.

5. **Place Grilled Salmon:**
   - Top the quinoa with grilled salmon fillets.

6. **Add Roasted Vegetables:**
   - Arrange the roasted veggies beside the salmon and quinoa.

7. **Serve and Enjoy:**
   - Your Grilled Salmon with Quinoa and Roasted Vegetables is ready to be enjoyed as a wholesome and delightful supper.

This recipe includes a well-rounded blend of omega-3 fatty acids from salmon, complete protein from quinoa, and a range of vitamins and minerals from roasted veggies. Customize the veggies and herbs depending on your tastes and enjoy a meal that improves your well-being.

Stuffed Bell Peppers with Lean Ground Turkey:

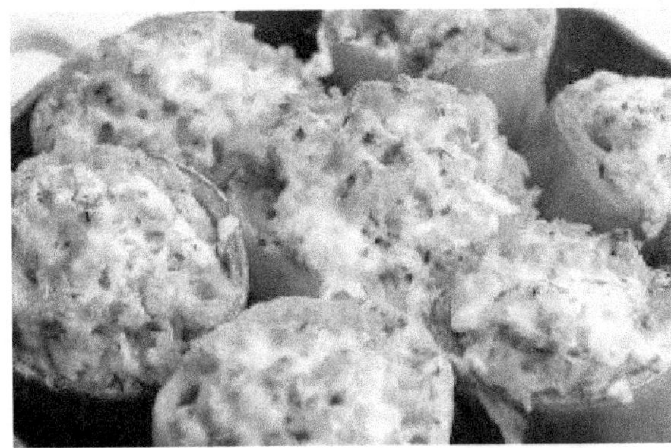

Ingredients:

For the Stuffed Bell Peppers:

- Bell peppers (assorted hues)
- Lean ground turkey
- Olive oil
- Onion, finely chopped Garlic, minced
- Cooked quinoa or brown rice
- Diced tomatoes (canned or fresh)
- Tomato sauce
- Ground cumin
- Paprika
- Salt and pepper

For Assembly:

- Grated cheese (such as mozzarella or cheddar)
- Fresh parsley or cilantro, chopped (for Garnish)

Instructions:

1. Prepare Bell Peppers:
   - Preheat the oven to 375°F (190°C).
   - Cut the tops off the bell peppers and remove the seeds and membranes.

2. Prepare Filling:
   - In a pan, heat olive oil over medium heat.
   - Add chopped onion and minced Garlic. Sauté until the onion is transparent.

3. Cook Ground Turkey:
   - Add lean ground turkey to the pan and sauté until browned and cooked.

4. Add Tomatoes and Spices:
   - Stir in chopped tomatoes, cooked quinoa or brown rice, tomato sauce, ground cumin, paprika, salt, salt, and pepper. Cook for a few minutes until the flavours merge.

5. Stuff Bell Peppers:
   - Place the hollowed-out bell peppers in a baking dish.
   - Fill each bell pepper with the turkey and rice mixture.

6. Bake:
   - Cover the baking dish with aluminium foil and bake in the oven for approximately 25-30 minutes or until the peppers are soft.

7. **Add Cheese and Finish Baking:**
   - Remove the foil and sprinkle grated cheese over the filled peppers.
   - Return the baking dish to the oven and bake for 5-7 minutes or until the cheese is melted and bubbling.

8. **Garnish and Serve:**
   - Garnish the filled bell peppers with chopped parsley or cilantro.

9. **Serve and Enjoy:**
   - Your Stuffed Bell Peppers with Lean Ground Turkey are ready to be enjoyed as a nutritious and fulfilling supper.

These filled bell peppers blend lean protein from ground turkey, fibre-rich quinoa or brown rice, and the natural sweetness of bell peppers. Customize the recipe with your preferred spices and herbs for a tasty supper that promotes adrenal health.

Vegetable Stir-Fry with Tofu:

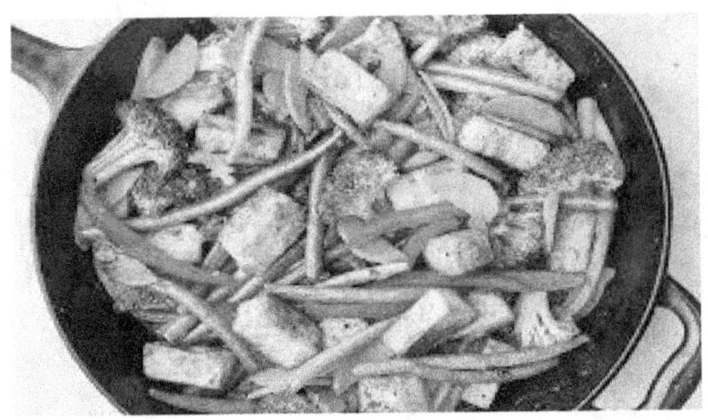

Ingredients:

For the Stir-Fry Sauce:
- Low-sodium soy sauce
- Vegetable broth or water
- Rice vinegar
- Hoisin sauce (optional)
- Cornstarch (to thicken)
- Ginger, minced Garlic, minced Red pepper flakes (optional)

For the Stir-Fry:
- Firm tofu, cubed
- Assorted vegetables (e.g., bell peppers, broccoli, snap peas, carrots), cut or chopped Olive oil or sesame oil
- Cooked brown rice or noodles

For Garnish:
- Sliced green onions
- Sesame seeds

Instructions:

1. **Prepare Stir-Fry Sauce:**
   - Mix low-sodium soy sauce, vegetable broth or water, rice vinegar, hoisin sauce (if used), cornstarch, minced Ginger, minced Garlic, and red pepper flakes (if used). Set aside.

2. **Stir-Fry Tofu:**
   - Heat a large skillet or wok over medium-high heat.
   - Add a drizzle of olive oil or sesame oil.
   - Add the cubed tofu and heat until gently browned and slightly crispy. Remove from the skillet and put aside.

3. **Stir-Fry Vegetables:**
   - In the same skillet, add a touch of extra oil if required.
   - Add the sliced or chopped veggies and stir-fry until they are tender-crisp.

4. **Add Tofu Back In:**
   - Return the cooked tofu to the skillet with the veggies.

5. **Add Stir-Fry Sauce:**
   - Pour the prepared stir-fry sauce over the tofu and veggies.

6. **Toss and Thicken:**
   - Toss everything together to ensure that the tofu and veggies are covered with the sauce.
   - Cook for a few minutes until the sauce thickens.

7. **Serve with Grains:**
   - Serve the vegetable and tofu stir-fry over cooked brown rice or noodles.

8. Garnish and Enjoy:
- Garnish the stir-fry with sliced green onions and sesame seeds for extra flavour and texture.

9. Serve and Enjoy:
- Your Vegetable Stir-Fry with Tofu is ready to be enjoyed as a tasty and plant-based meal.

This stir-fry gives a flash of colour, taste, and nutrition from various veggies and protein-packed tofu. The flavorful stir-fry sauce combines all the components for a fulfilling dinner, promoting adrenal health. Customize the veggies and change the degree of spiciness to your desire.

Baked Chicken with Sweet Potato and Asparagus:

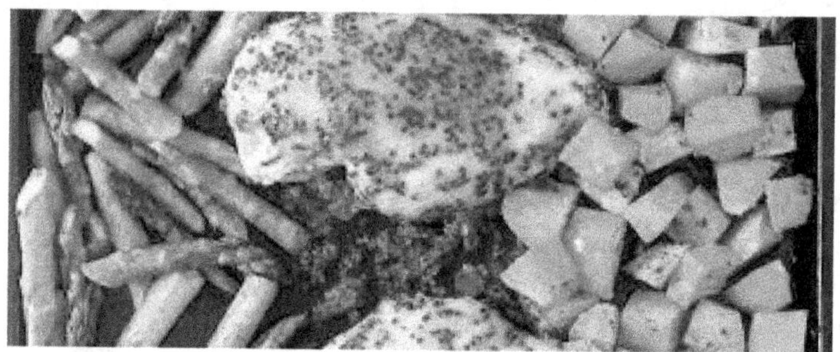

Ingredients:

For the Baked Chicken:
- Chicken breasts or thighs
- Olive oil Garlic powder

- Paprika
- Salt and pepper

For the Sweet Potatoes:
- Sweet potatoes, peeled and diced Olive oil
- Ground cumin
- Smoked paprika
- Salt and pepper

For the Asparagus:
- Fresh asparagus spears, trimmed Olive oil
- Lemon zest, SaltSalt & pepper

Instructions:

1. **Preheat the Oven:**
   - Preheat the oven to 400°F (200°C).

2. **Prepare Baked Chicken:**
   - Rub the chicken breasts or thighs with olive oil.
   - Season both sides of the chicken with garlic powder, paprika, salt, salt, and pepper.

3. **Prepare Sweet Potatoes:**
   - Combine diced sweet potatoes with olive oil, ground cumin, smoked paprika, salt, salt, and pepper in a bowl.

4. **Arrange on Baking Sheet:**
    - Place the seasoned chicken on one side of a baking sheet.
    - Spread the seasoned sweet potatoes on the opposite side of the baking sheet.

5. **Bake:**
    - Place the baking sheet in the oven and bake for approximately 20-25 minutes, until the chicken is cooked and the sweet potatoes are soft.

6. **Prepare Asparagus:**
    - Combine trimmed asparagus spears in another dish with olive oil, lemon zest, salt, salt, and pepper.

7. **Add Asparagus to Baking Sheet:**
    - After baking for 10-15 minutes, put the prepped asparagus on the oven sheet with the chicken and sweet potatoes.

8. **Continue Baking:**
    - Continue baking for 10-15 minutes or until the asparagus is tender and slightly crunchy.

9. **Serve and Enjoy:**
    - Your Baked Chicken with Sweet Potato and Asparagus is ready to be enjoyed as a nutritious and pleasant supper.

This recipe includes lean protein from chicken, complex carbs from sweet potatoes, and fibre-rich minerals from asparagus.

The mix of tastes and textures provides a balanced meal promoting adrenal health. Customize the seasoning and cooking times depending on your preferences for a customized gourmet experience.

Lentil and Vegetable Curry:

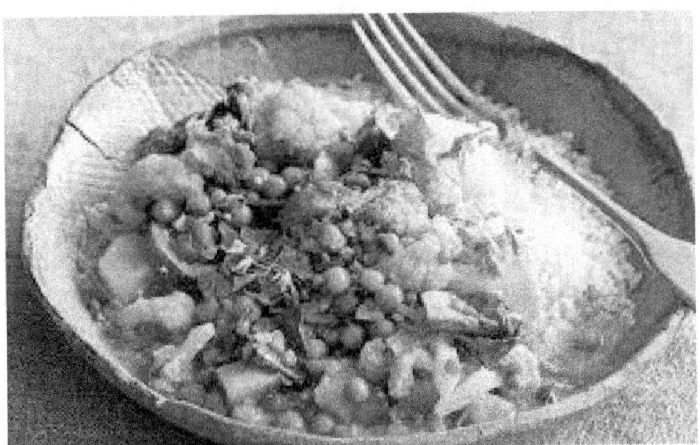

Ingredients:

For the Curry Sauce:

- Onion, chopped Garlic, minced Ginger, minced Curry powder
- Ground turmeric
- Ground cumin
- Ground coriander
- Tomato paste
- Coconut milk
- Vegetable broth
- Salt and pepper

For the Lentil and Vegetable Curry:

- Green or brown lentils, washed and drained
- Assorted veggies (e.g., carrots, bell peppers, cauliflower, peas), chopped Olive oil or cooking oil of choice
- Fresh cilantro leaves, chopped (for Garnish)

Instructions:

1. Prepare Curry Sauce:
   - In a large skillet or saucepan, heat olive oil over medium heat.
   - Add chopped onion and sauté until transparent.
   - Add minced Garlic and minced Ginger, and sauté for approximately 1 minute until fragrant.

2. Add Spices and Tomato Paste:
   - Stir in curry powder, powdered turmeric, ground cumin, coriander, and tomato paste.
   - Cook for a few minutes to roast the spices and combine the flavours.

3. Add Coconut Milk and Vegetable Broth:
   - Pour in coconut milk and vegetable broth.
   - Stir well to blend the ingredients and bring the mixture to a boil.

4. Add Lentils and Vegetables:
   - Add washed lentils and chopped veggies to the curry sauce.
   - Stir to coat the lentils and veggies with the sauce.

- Simmer and Cook

- Cover the pan or pot and let the curry simmer over medium-low heat for approximately 20-25 minutes or until the lentils and veggies are cooked.

5. **Season and Garnish:**
   - Season the curry with SaltSalt and pepper to taste.
   - Garnish with chopped fresh cilantro leaves before serving.

6. **Serve and Enjoy:**
   - Your Lentil and Vegetable Curry is ready to be enjoyed as a beautiful and healthy supper.

This curry delivers a delicious balance of protein from lentils and vitamins and minerals from colourful veggies. The fragrant spices provide depth of flavour, making this dish a soothing option for a balanced meal promoting adrenal health. Serve the curry over cooked brown rice or whole-grain couscous for a complete and hearty supper.

Zucchini Noodles with Tomato Sauce and Grilled Chicken:

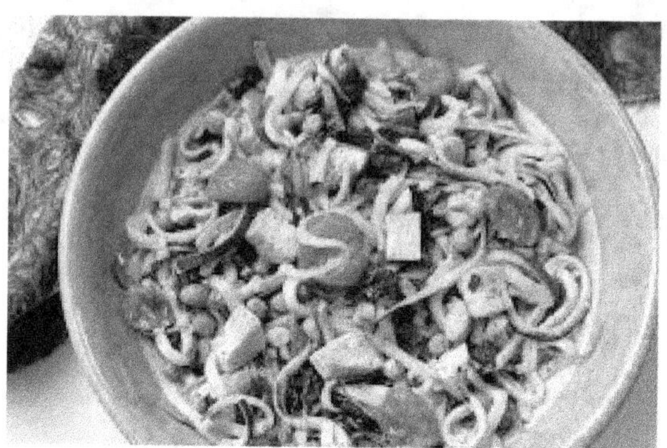

Ingredients:

For the Grilled Chicken:

- Chicken breasts or thighs
- Olive oil Italian seasoning (or a blend of dried basil, oregano, and thyme)
- Salt and pepper

For the Zucchini Noodles:

- Zucchini spiralized into noodles
- Olive oil
- Garlic, minced
- Red pepper flakes (optional)
- Salt and pepper

For the Tomato Sauce:

- Canned crushed tomatoes
- Garlic, minced
- Dried basil
- Dried oregano
- Salt and pepper

Instructions:

1. **Prepare Grilled Chicken:**
   - Rub the chicken breasts or thighs with olive oil.
   - Season both sides with Italian seasoning, salt, salt, and pepper.
   - Grill the chicken until thoroughly done, approximately 6-8 minutes each side. Once done, let it rest before slicing.

2. **Prepare Zucchini Noodles:**
   - In a pan, heat olive oil over medium heat.
   - Add minced Garlic and red pepper flakes (if using) and sauté for approximately 1 minute until aromatic.
   - Add spiralized zucchini noodles and sauté for a few minutes until soft but still somewhat crunchy.
   - Season with salt, salt, and pepper to taste.

3. **Make Tomato Sauce:**
   - In a separate saucepan, heat a little olive oil over medium heat.
   - Add minced Garlic and simmer for approximately 1 minute until fragrant.

- Stir in canned crushed tomatoes, dried basil, dry oregano, salt, salt, and pepper.
- Let the sauce boil for a few minutes to combine the flavours.

4. **Assemble the Dish:**
   - Arrange a piece of zucchini noodles on each dish.

5. **Add Tomato Sauce and Chicken:**
   - Spoon tomato sauce over the zucchini noodles.
   - Top with sliced grilled chicken.

6. **Serve and Enjoy:**
   - Your Zucchini Noodles with Tomato Sauce and Grilled Chicken are ready to be enjoyed as a light and savoury meal.

This meal provides a low-carb alternative to classic pasta by mixing zucchini noodles with a rich tomato sauce and protein-packed grilled chicken. Customize the ingredients and alter the amount of spiciness to your preference. It's a tasty and adrenal health-supportive supper acceptable for people seeking a gluten-free alternative.

Mediterranean Chickpea Salad with Feta:

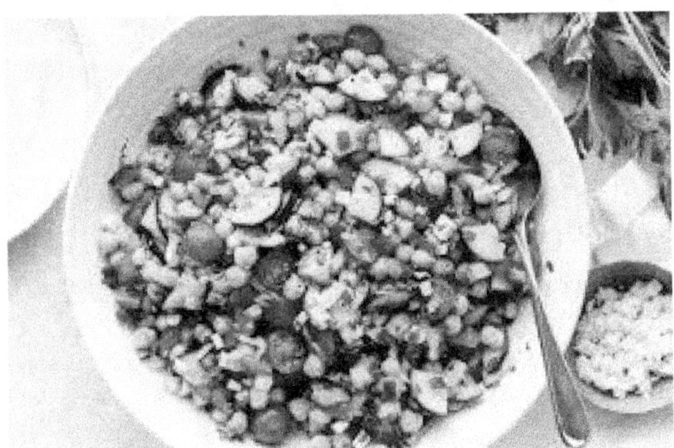

Ingredients:

For the Salad:

- Canned chickpeas,
- drained and rinsed Cucumber,
- diced Cherry tomatoes,
- halved Red onion,
- finely chopped Kalamata olives,
- pitted and halved Fresh parsley,
- chopped Feta cheese,
- crumbled

For the Dressing:

- Olive oil
- Lemon juice
- Red wine vinegar
- Garlic, minced

- Dried oregano
- Salt and pepper

Instructions:

1. **Prepare Chickpea Salad:**
   - Add the canned chickpeas, sliced Cucumber, half cherry tomatoes, finely chopped red onion, halved Kalamata olives, chopped fresh parsley, and crumbled feta cheese in a large bowl.

2. **Prepare Dressing:**
   - Mix olive oil, lemon juice, red wine vinegar, minced Garlic, dried oregano, salt, salt, and pepper to produce the dressing in a separate dish.

3. **Assemble the Salad:**
   - Pour the dressing over the chickpea mixture.

4. **Toss and Combine:**
   - Mix all the ingredients until thoroughly blended and uniformly covered with the dressing.

5. **Adjust Seasonings:**
   - Taste the salad and adjust the spices if required by adding more salt, pepper, or lemon juice.

6. **Chill and Marinate:**
   - Cover the salad and let it rest in the refrigerator for at least 30 minutes to enable the flavours to mingle.

7. Serve and Enjoy:
   - Your Mediterranean Chickpea Salad with Feta is ready to be enjoyed as a light and tasty meal.

This salad combines the richness of protein-rich chickpeas, fresh veggies, and tangy feta cheese, all accentuated by the Mediterranean-inspired dressing. It's an excellent alternative for a fast and nutrient-packed lunch that promotes adrenal health. Feel free to add additional such as chopped fresh mint, sliced bell peppers, or artichoke hearts for extra tastes and textures.

Quinoa and Black Bean Bowl with Avocado:

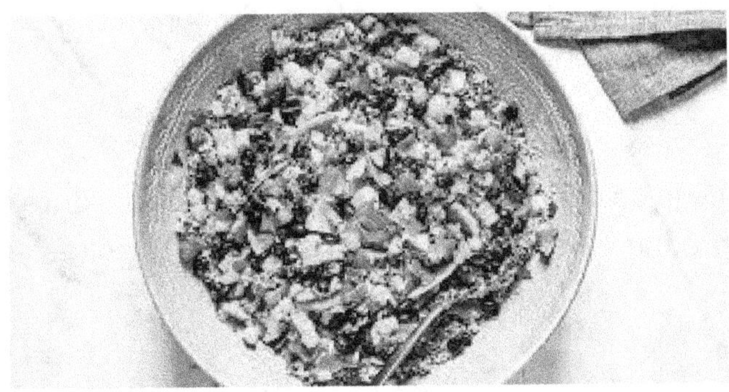

Ingredients:

For the Quinoa and Black Bean Bowl:
   - Cooked quinoa
   - Cooked black beans (canned or cooked from dry)
   - Red onion, finely chopped
   - Red bell pepper, diced

- Corn kernels (fresh, frozen, or canned)
- Fresh cilantro, chopped Lime juice
- Ground cumin
- Salt and pepper

For Assembly:
- Ripe avocados,
- sliced Lime wedges

Instructions:

1. Prepare Quinoa and Black Bean Bowl:
   - Add cooked quinoa, black beans, finely sliced red onion, diced red bell pepper, corn kernels, and chopped fresh cilantro in a large bowl.

2. Season and Toss:
   - Drizzle lime juice over the quinoa and black bean mixture.
   - Sprinkle ground cumin, salt, salt, and pepper to taste.
   - Gently mix all the ingredients to disperse the flavours.

3. Assemble the Bowl:
   - Divide the quinoa and black bean mixture into serving dishes.

4. Add Avocado Slices:
   - Top each dish with slices of ripe avocado.

5. **Squeeze Lime:**
   - Squeeze fresh lime juice over the avocado slices.

6. **Serve and Enjoy:**
   - Your Quinoa and Black Bean Bowl with Avocado is ready to be enjoyed as a tasty and nutrient-rich supper.

This dish delivers a mix of protein from the quinoa and black beans, fibre from veggies, and the creamy deliciousness of avocado. The lime juice and ground cumin give the meal a refreshing and zesty taste. Customize the ingredients according to your preferences, and feel free to add extras like diced tomatoes, chopped green onions, or a splash of spicy sauce for added spice. It's a diverse and adrenal health-supportive dish that's simple to make and enjoy.

Baked Cod with Roasted Brussels Sprouts and Quinoa:

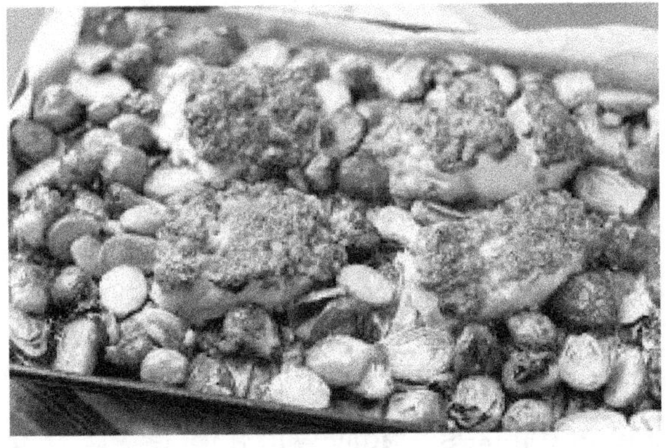

Ingredients:

For the Baked Cod:
- Cod fillets
- Olive oil
- Lemon juice
- Fresh herbs (such as thyme or dill)
- Salt and pepper

For the Roasted Brussels Sprouts:
- Brussels sprouts, cut and halved
- Olive oil
- Balsamic vinegar
- Garlic powder
- Salt and pepper

For the Quinoa:
- Quinoa Vegetable broth or water Salt

Instructions:

1. Prepare Baked Cod:
- Preheat the oven to 400°F (200°C).
- Place the fish fillets on a baking pan lined with parchment paper.
- Drizzle olive oil and lemon juice over the fillets.
- Sprinkle fresh herbs, salt, and pepper to taste.
- Bake in the oven for approximately 12-15 minutes or until the cod is opaque and flakes readily with a fork.

2. **Prepare Roasted Brussels Sprouts:**
   - Combine halved Brussels sprouts in a bowl with olive oil, balsamic vinegar, garlic powder, salt, and pepper.
   - Spread the Brussels sprouts on a separate baking sheet in a single layer.
   - Roast in the oven for approximately 20-25 minutes or until the Brussels sprouts are caramelized and soft.

3. **Prepare Quinoa:**
   - Rinse the quinoa well in cold water.
   - In a saucepan, blend quinoa and vegetable broth (or water) in a 2:1 ratio (2 parts liquid to 1 part quinoa).
   - Add a pinch of salt and bring to a boil. Reduce heat, cover, and simmer for approximately 15-20 minutes, or until the quinoa is cooked and the liquid is absorbed.

4. **Assemble the Dish:**
   - Arrange a bed of cooked quinoa on each serving platter.
   - Place Baked Cod and Roasted Brussels Sprouts:

   - Place a cooked fish fillet on the bed of quinoa.
   - Add a portion of roasted Brussels sprouts beside the fish.

5. **Serve and Enjoy:**
   - Your Baked Cod with Roasted Brussels Sprouts and Quinoa is ready to be enjoyed as a nutritious and delightful supper.

This recipe delivers a mix of protein from the fish, Brussels sprouts fibre and quinoa complex carbs. The roasted Brussels sprouts offer a great crunch and depth of flavour. Customize the herbs and spices to your preference, and enjoy a meal that promotes adrenal health and delivers a well-rounded mix of nutrients.

Turkey and Vegetable Stir-Fry:

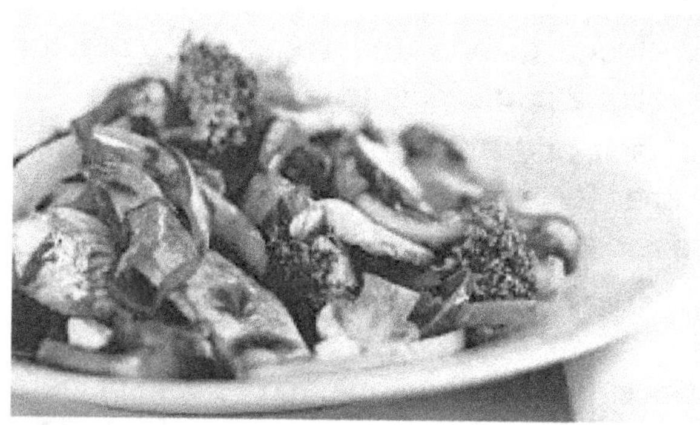

Ingredients:

For the Stir-Fry Sauce:
- Low-sodium soy sauce
- Hoisin sauce (optional)
- Rice vinegar
- Sesame oil
- Cornstarch (to thicken)
- Ginger, minced
- Garlic, minced
- Red pepper flakes (optional)

For the Stir-Fry:

- Ground turkey
- Assorted veggies (e.g., bell peppers, broccoli, snap peas, carrots), sliced or chopped Olive or sesame oil.

For Serving:

- Cooked brown rice or whole-grain noodles
- Sliced green onions
- Sesame seeds

Instructions:

1. Prepare Stir-Fry Sauce:
   - Mix low-sodium soy sauce, hoisin sauce (if used), rice vinegar, sesame oil, cornstarch, chopped ginger, minced garlic, and red pepper flakes (if used). Set aside.

2. Cook Ground Turkey:
   - Heat a dab of olive oil or sesame oil over medium-high heat in a big skillet or wok.
   - Add ground turkey and heat until browned and cooked through. Break up the turkey into smaller pieces while it cooks.

3. Add Vegetables:\
   - Push the cooked turkey to one side of the pan and add more oil to the other.
   - Add the sliced or chopped veggies to the pan and stir-fry until tender-crisp.

4. **Combine with Sauce:**
   - Push the veggies to one side of the pan and pour the prepared stir-fry sauce into the cleared space.
   - Stir the sauce until it thickens and coats the back of a spoon.

5. **Mix Everything:**
   - Combine the cooked ground turkey and stir-fried veggies with the thickened sauce.

6. **Serve with Grains:**
   - Serve the turkey and veggie stir-fry over cooked brown rice or whole-grain noodles.

7. **Garnish and Enjoy:**
   - Garnish the stir-fry with sliced green onions and sesame seeds for extra flavour and texture.

8. **Serve and Enjoy:**
   - Your Turkey and Vegetable Stir-Fry is ready to be enjoyed as a tasty and balanced supper.

This stir-fry blends the lean protein of ground turkey with a mix of colourful veggies and a flavorful sauce. It's a flexible dish that enables you to use your favourite vegetables and modify the amount of spice. Serve it over your choice of nutritious grains for a balanced and fulfilling dinner that promotes adrenal health.

CHAPTER SEVEN

Healing Beverages

Herbal Teas

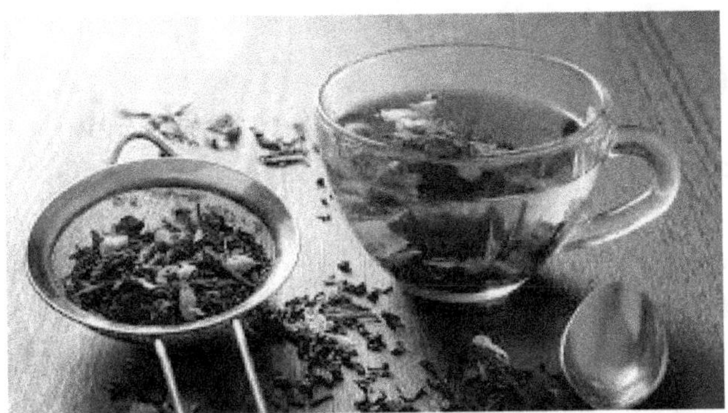

Herbal teas are an excellent alternative to enhance adrenal health and general well-being. Here are some herbal teas that you may add to your routine:

1. **Chamomile Tea:**
   Chamomile is recognized for its relaxing and soothing effects. It may assist in inducing relaxation and improved sleep, which can be suitable for controlling stress.

2. **Peppermint Tea:**
   Peppermint tea has a pleasant taste and may help reduce intestinal pain, which may be aggravated by stress.

3. **Lemon Balm Tea:**

   Lemon balm is a benign plant with modest sedative effects. It's typically used to improve relaxation and ease anxiety.

4. **Passionflower Tea:**

   Passionflower is recognized for its relaxing qualities and may help alleviate uneasiness and restlessness.

5. **Valerian Root Tea:**

   Valerian root is known to have relaxing effects and may assist in enhancing sleep quality and lowering anxiety.

6. **Lavender Tea:**

   Lavender is recognized for its relaxing perfume, and drinking lavender tea may help quiet the mind and generate a feeling of serenity.

7. **Licorice Root Tea:**

   Liquorice root is an adaptogenic plant that may assist in maintaining adrenal function and regulating cortisol levels.

8. **Holy Basil (Tulsi) Tea:**

   Holy basil, commonly known as Tulsi, is an adaptogenic plant that may help the body adapt to stress and enhance general well-being.

9. **Nettle Tea:**

   Nettle tea is rich in vitamins and minerals, making it a healthy option that may help promote overall health.

Hibiscus tea is tasty and rich in antioxidants that may improve heart health and prevent oxidative stress.

When picking herbal teas, consider your particular tastes and any possible allergies or conflicts with drugs. Herbal teas may be a peaceful and delightful method to introduce beneficial herbs into your daily routine to promote adrenal health and general relaxation.

Green Tea Green Tea is a popular beverage with several health advantages, including possible support for adrenal function. Here's why green Tea might be an intelligent option for increasing general wellbeing:

- **Rich in Antioxidants:** Green Tea contains antioxidants, such as catechins and polyphenols, which help counteract oxidative stress and decrease inflammation. These antioxidants help to a healthy body and enhance adrenal function.

- **L-Theanine Content:** Green Tea includes an amino acid called L-theanine, which has been found to have relaxing and stress-reducing properties. L-theanine may induce relaxation without inducing sleepiness, making green Tea a suitable alternative for reducing stress.

- **Caffeine concentration:** While green Tea contains caffeine, the caffeine concentration is often lower than coffee's. This modest dose of caffeine may offer a pleasant energy boost without generating significant jitters or adrenal strain.

- **Metabolism Support:** Some studies show that the combination of catechins and caffeine in green Tea has a good impact on metabolism and fat oxidation, which helps with weight control.

- **Heart Health:** Green Tea may enhance cardiovascular health by helping to reduce cholesterol levels, boosting

Blood artery function, and lowering the risk of heart disease.

- **Brain Health:** The combination of L-theanine and caffeine in green Tea may have synergistic benefits on cognitive function, including greater attention, alertness, and mental clarity.

- **Antibacterial qualities:** Green Tea contains natural antibacterial qualities, which may assist in promoting a healthy immune system.

When sipping green Tea, here are a few tips:

- **Choose High-Quality Tea:** Opt for high-quality loose-leaf green Tea or high-grade tea bags to guarantee the finest taste and health benefits.

- **Brewing:** Brew green tea with water slightly below boiling (about 175°F or 80°C) to prevent bitterness. Steep for roughly 2-3 minutes.

- **Types:** There are several types of green Tea, including sencha, matcha, and genmaicha. Each has its distinct taste profile and advantages.

- **Moderation:** While green Tea is usually considered safe, eating it in moderation is vital, particularly if you're sensitive to caffeine.

As usual, it's a good idea to talk with a healthcare practitioner, particularly if you have any underlying health concerns or are taking medicines, before changing your diet or beverage choices.

Ginger Turmeric Latte (Golden Milk):

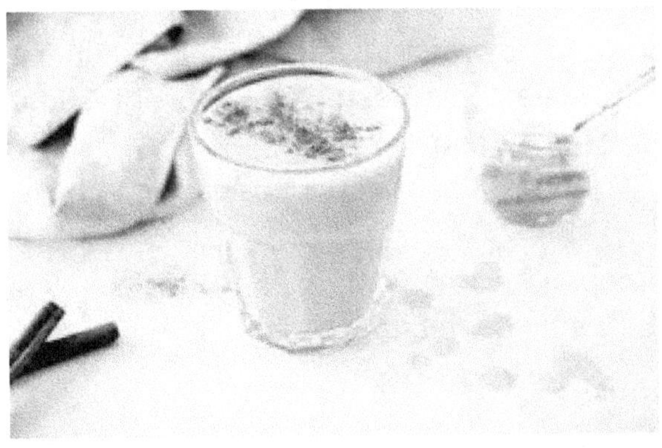

Ingredients:

For the Turmeric Paste (optional but recommended):

Turmeric powder Water For the Latte:
- Milk of your choosing (dairy, almond, coconut, etc.)
- Fresh ginger, grated or minced
- Ground turmeric
- Ground cinnamon
- Ground black pepper
- Honey or sweetener of choice (optional)
- Coconut oil or ghee (clarified butter) for extra creaminess (optional)

Instructions:

1. Prepare Turmeric Paste (Optional but Recommended):
   - In a small saucepan, blend turmeric powder and water to produce a paste. Use around 1/4 cup of turmeric powder to 1/2 cup of water.
   - Heat the mixture over low heat, stirring regularly, until it becomes a thick paste. This paste may be kept in the refrigerator for a week or two.

2. Prepare Latte:
   - In a small saucepan, warm your milk of choice over medium heat. Be cautious not to cook it.

3. **Add Ginger and Turmeric:**
    - Add freshly grated or chopped ginger to the heated milk.
    - Add a pinch of ground turmeric, cinnamon, and a tiny amount of ground black pepper. The black pepper helps improve the absorption of curcumin, the critical component of turmeric.

4. **Add Sweetener and Coconut Oil/Ghee:**
    - If desired, add honey or a sweetener of your choice to taste.
    - Try adding a little quantity of coconut oil or ghee for additional creaminess.

5. **Stir and Warm:**
    - Stir the mixture carefully to incorporate all the ingredients.
    - Heat the mixture gradually, stirring regularly, until it's warm but not boiling.

6. **Strain and Serve:**
    - If preferred, sieve the mixture to remove any ginger fragments.
    - Pour the Ginger Turmeric Latte into a cup.

7. **Enjoy:**
    - Your Ginger Turmeric Latte is ready to be enjoyed as a pleasant and health-supportive drink.

Golden Milk delivers the anti-inflammatory effects of turmeric and the relaxing characteristics of ginger, making it a popular option for improving general well-being and assisting in relaxation.

Customize the flavours and sweetness to your preference and appreciate this latte's warm and fragrant pleasure. Integrating these potent substances into your everyday routine is a terrific approach.

Lemon Balm Tea

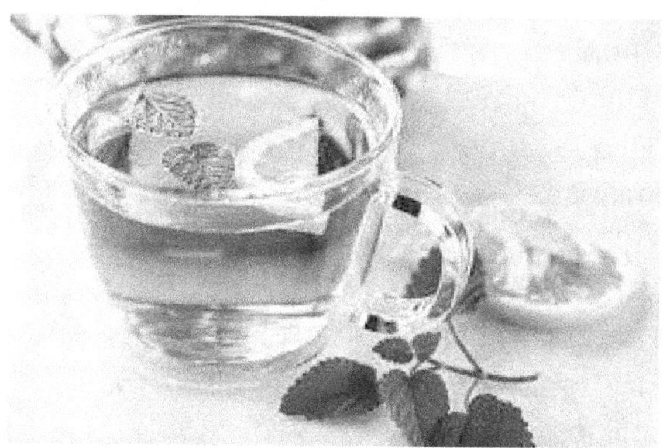

Ingredients:

- Fresh lemon balm leaves (approximately one tablespoon of mint leaves per cup) OR Dried lemon balm leaves (about one teaspoon of dried leaves per cup)
- Boiling water

Instructions:

1. Harvest or Obtain Lemon Balm Leaves:
   - You may gather fresh leaves if you have access to a lemon balm plant. Otherwise, you may get dried lemon balm leaves at health food shops or online.

2. **Prepare the Leaves:**
   - If using fresh leaves, wash them carefully and remove any stems.
   - If using dried leaves, measure the quantity of the cups you wish to brew.

3. **Boil Water:**
   - Heat water to a boil in a kettle or saucepan. You'll need enough water to fill your teacup or teapot.

4. **Place Lemon Balm Leaves in a Teapot or Cup:**
   - Add the fresh or dried lemon balm leaves to your teapot or straight into a cup or mug.

5. **Pour Boiling Water:**
   - Carefully pour the boiling water over the lemon balm leaves.

6. **Steep:**
   - Cover the teapot or cup with a cover or saucer to contain the steam and scent.
   - Let the lemon balm soak for 5-10 minutes to extract the flavour and benefits.

7. **Strain (Optional):**
   - If you use loose-leaf lemon balm, you may filter the Tea into another cup to remove the leaves. If you used a teabag or an infuser, remove it.

8. Enjoy:
   - Sip your lemon balm tea gently and experience its delicate, lemony taste and relaxing effects.

Lemon balm tea is noted for its possible advantages, including:

   - **Calming Effect:** Lemon balm is widely used to induce relaxation and relieve tension and anxiety.

   - **Digestive Aid:** It may help alleviate digestive pain and treat moderate indigestion.

   - **Improved Sleep:** Some individuals find that lemon balm tea may assist in enhancing sleep quality and decreasing restlessness.

   - **Antioxidant Properties:** Lemon balm includes antioxidants that may help general health.

   - **Modest Antiviral qualities:** It's been used historically for its subtle antiviral attributes.

Lemon balm tea is caffeine-free and usually considered harmless. It's a delightful and caffeine-free alternative for a tranquil and soothing beverage.

Ashwagandha Elixir

Ingredients:

- Ashwagandha powder or extract (see package recommendations for dosing)
- Warm water or milk of your choice (dairy, almond, coconut, etc.)
- Honey or sweetener of choice (optional)
- Ground cardamom, cinnamon, or nutmeg (for taste, optional)

Instructions:

1. Measure Ashwagandha:
   - Start by measuring the required dose of ashwagandha powder or extract. Follow the recommendations on the product label since quantities may vary.

2. Warm Water or Milk:
   - Heat your choice of warm water or milk in a pot. Avoid boiling; only heat until it's warm.

3. Mix Ashwagandha:
   - Add the measured ashwagandha powder or extract to the heated drink. Stir thoroughly to dissolve it.

4. Add Sweetener and Flavor (Optional):
   - Add a drizzle of honey or your favourite sweetener for flavour if desired.

- Add a sprinkle of ground cardamom, cinnamon, or nutmeg for flavour.

5. **Stir and Enjoy:**
    - Stir the elixir carefully to ensure the ashwagandha is well blended.
    - Sip your Ashwagandha Elixir gently and appreciate its possible benefits.

Important Considerations:

- **Dose:** Always follow the prescribed dose directions on the ashwagandha product packaging. Consult a healthcare expert before using, particularly if you have any underlying health concerns or are taking drugs.

- **Pregnancy and Lactation:** Pregnant and breastfeeding persons should see their healthcare professional before consuming ashwagandha.

- **Flavour Preferences:** Feel free to personalize the elixir to your taste preferences. You may vary the quantity of sugar and flavourings to suit your preferences.

Ashwagandha is considered to provide potential advantages, which include stress reduction, increased sleep quality, and boosting general well-being. However, individual reactions may differ. If you're contemplating introducing ashwagandha into your routine, you should check with a healthcare practitioner to confirm it's suitable for your health requirements.

Beet Juice

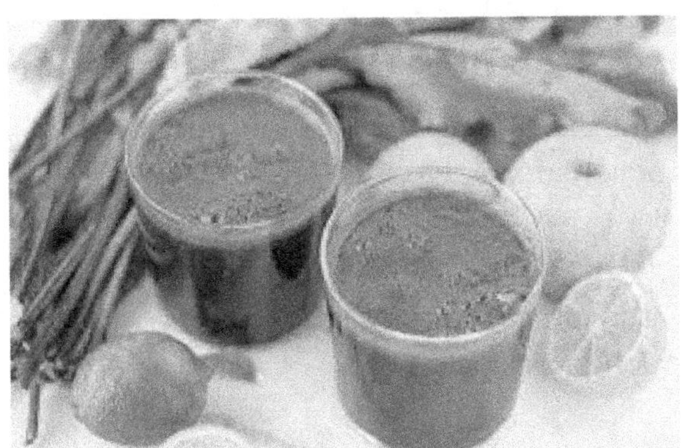

Ingredients:

- Fresh beets (typically 1-2 medium-sized beets)
- Lemon juice (optional, for taste)
- Water (for diluting, if required)
- Sweetener (optional)
- Ice cubes (optional)

Instructions:

1. Prepare Beets:
   - Wash and clean the beets carefully to eliminate any dirt.
   - Remove the tops and tails of the beets.

2. Peel and Cut:
   - Depending on your juicer's capacity and choice, you may peel the beets or leave the skin on. Be cautious to remove any rough or blemished areas.

- Cut the beets into smaller pieces that suit your juicer's feed tube.

3. Juice the Beets:
   - Use a juicer to extract the juice from the beets. Follow your juicer's directions for optimal results.

4. Add Lemon Juice (Optional):
   - Add a dash of fresh lemon juice to the beet juice for extra flavour and a touch of acidity.

5. Dilute (Optional):
   - Beet juice may be potent, so you can dilute it with water to your chosen strength.

6. Add Sweetener (Optional):
   - If you find the flavour of pure beet juice too harsh, you may add a natural sweetener like honey or agave syrup to taste.

7. Chill or Serve Over Ice:
   - You may refrigerate the beet juice to cool it or pour it over ice for a pleasant cocktail.

8. Enjoy:
   - Sip your beet juice carefully and relish its earthy and slightly sweet taste.

9. Important Considerations:

- **Staining:** Beets are recognized for their bright red hue, which may stain surfaces and clothes. Be careful when handling them.

- **Potential Benefits:** Beet juice is high in dietary nitrates, which may assist in enhancing blood flow and workout performance. It also includes antioxidants and other minerals.

- **Digestive System:** Be warned that ingesting a large quantity of beet juice in one sitting might produce transitory changes in urine and stool colour owing to the pigment called betacyanin.

Beet juice may be drunk alone or blended with other fruits and vegetables to produce tasty, nutrient-packed drinks. It's a pleasant and health-supportive beverage that may be part of a balanced diet.

CHAPTER EIGHT

Adrenal-Supportive Sweets

Dark Chocolate-Dipped Berries

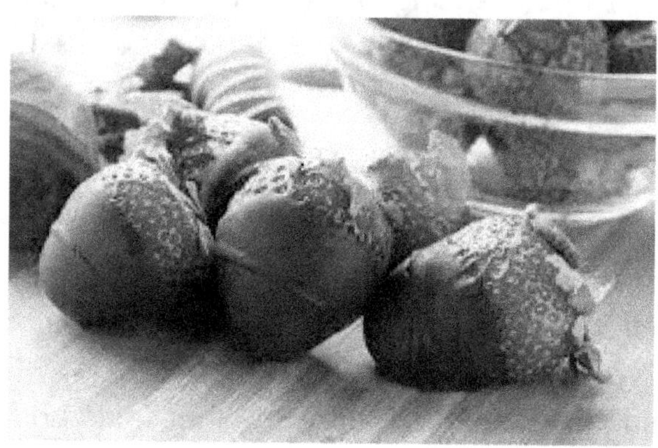

Ingredients:

- Fresh berries (such as strawberries, blueberries, raspberries, or blackberries)
- Dark chocolate (70% cocoa or more significant)
- Optional toppings (chopped almonds, shredded coconut, sea salt, etc.)

Instructions:

1. Prepare Berries:
   - Wash and carefully wipe dry the berries to eliminate any moisture. Make sure they are thoroughly dry before dipping them in chocolate.

2. **Melt Dark Chocolate:**
   - Break the dark chocolate into tiny pieces and set them in a microwave-safe basin, or use a double boiler to melt the chocolate. If using a microwave, heat in 20-second intervals, stirring between intervals until the chocolate is melted.

3. **Dip Berries:**
   - Hold each berry by its stem or a toothpick and dip it into the melted dark chocolate. Swirl to cover the fruit half or fully, as desired.

4. **Drain Excess Chocolate:**
   - Allow any extra chocolate to trickle back into the dish.

5. **Optional Toppings:**
   - While the chocolate is still wet, sprinkle chopped almonds, shredded coconut, or sea salt over the dipped berries for extra taste and texture.

6. **Place on Parchment Paper:**
   - Place the dipped berries on a parchment paper-lined tray to cool and set.

7. **Cool and Set:**
   - Allow the chocolate-dipped berries to cool and the chocolate to set fully. You may speed up the process by putting them in the refrigerator for a short period.

8. Serve and Enjoy:
   - Once the chocolate is solid, your Dark Chocolate-Dipped Berries are ready to be savoured. Serve them as a delicious snack or a nutritious dessert.

Dark chocolate includes antioxidants and may offer possible health advantages when taken in moderation. Like strawberries and blueberries, Berries are also high in vitamins, fibre, and antioxidants. This combination creates a treat that's tasty and delivers some nutritious benefits. Remember to buy high-quality dark chocolate with a high cocoa content for the most incredible taste and health benefits.

Date Energy Balls

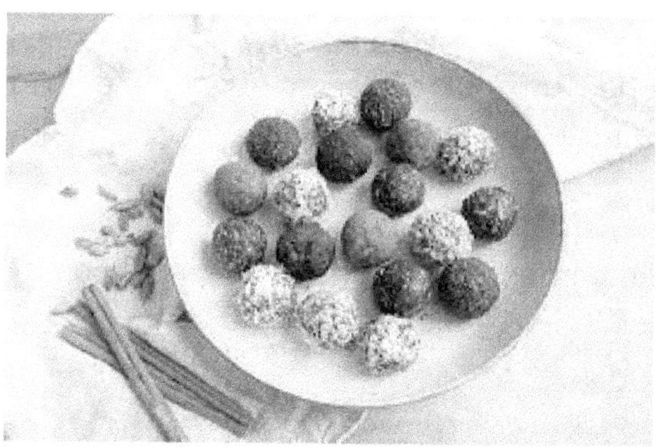

Ingredients:
   - Medjool dates (pitted)
   - Nuts (such as almonds, cashews, walnuts)
   - Unsweetened shredded coconut

- Natural nut butter (almond, peanut, cashew, etc.)
- Optional add-ins (cocoa powder, chia seeds, vanilla extract, etc.)
- Optional toppings (coconut flakes, crushed almonds, cocoa powder, etc.)

Instructions:

1. **Prepare Dates and Nuts:**
   - If the dates are not soft, soak them in warm water for approximately 10 minutes to soften. Drain the water before using.
   - If using whole nuts, you may toast them briefly in a dry pan over medium heat for extra flavour.

2. **Blend Dates and Nuts:**
   - In a food processor, mix the pitted dates and nuts. Process until they create a sticky and crumbly mixture.

3. **Add Nut Butter and Flavorings:**
   - Add a teaspoon of natural nut butter and desired flavourings, such as vanilla extract or chocolate powder, to the processor.

4. **Blend Until Combined:**
   - Process the ingredients again until everything is fully incorporated, producing a dough-like consistency.

5. **Add Shredded Coconut:**
   - Add some unsweetened shredded coconut to the mixture and pulse quickly to integrate.
6. **Form Balls:**
   - Roll a tiny quantity of the mixture between your hands to create bite-sized balls.

7. **Add Toppings (Optional):**
   - Roll the balls in toppings like coconut flakes, chopped almonds, or cocoa powder for extra texture and taste.

8. **Chill:**
   - Place the energy balls on a dish lined with parchment paper and chill them in the refrigerator for at least 30 minutes to solidify.

9. **Store and Enjoy:**
   - Once set, transfer the date energy balls to an airtight container. They may be kept in the refrigerator for up to two weeks.

10. **Grab and Go:**
    - Enjoy these energy balls as a fast and healthful snack anytime you need a burst of energy.

Date energy balls are a terrific source of natural sweetness, fibre, healthy fats, and energy-boosting elements. They're great for fulfilling your sweet cravings while giving continuous energy. Customize the ingredients and flavours of your choice and enjoy these delightful and nutrient-packed snacks.

Baked Apple with Cinnamon

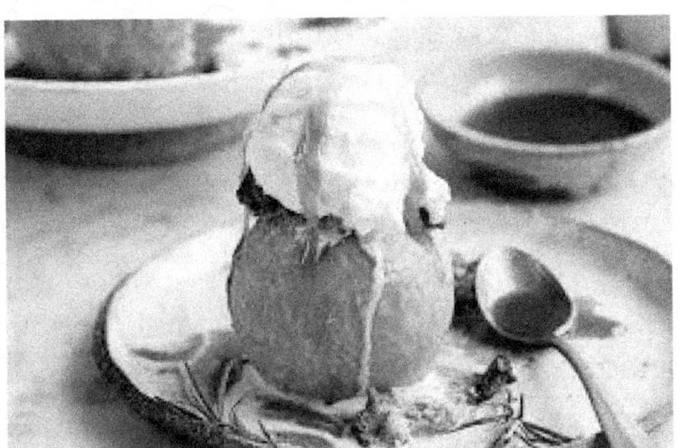

Ingredients:

- Apples (such as Granny Smith, Honeycrisp, or Fuji)
- Ground cinnamon
- Optional toppings (chopped nuts, raisins, a sprinkle of honey, etc.)

Instructions:

1. Preheat the Oven:
   - Preheat your oven to 375°F (190°C).

2. Prepare Apples:
   - Wash and core the apples. You may leave the skin on for additional nutrients and texture.
3. Spice the Apples:
   - Sprinkle ground cinnamon over the apples. Use as much or as little as you desire, depending on your taste.

4. **Optional Toppings:**
   - Add toppings like chopped nuts (such as walnuts or almonds) and a few raisins for added taste and texture.

5. **Bake the Apples:**
   - Place the spiced apples in a baking dish. If the apples have a hollow core from coring, you may fill them with some toppings.
   - Bake the apples in the oven for approximately 20-30 minutes or until they are soft when pricked with a fork.

6. **Serve Warm:**
   - Remove the roasted apples from the oven and allow them to cool slightly.
   - Serve the baked apples warm as a cosy and naturally sweet dessert.

7. **Enjoy:**
   - Enjoy the delightful blend of baked apples and cinnamon. You may eat them as is or add a dollop of yoghurt, a drizzle of honey, or a sprinkle of more cinnamon for added flavour.

Baked apples are a healthier alternative to classic sweets since they don't need extra sugars. They're rich in fibre, vitamins, and antioxidants. This delight is excellent for fall or whenever you're seeking a warm and cosy dessert without extra sweetness.

Homemade Fruit Sorbet

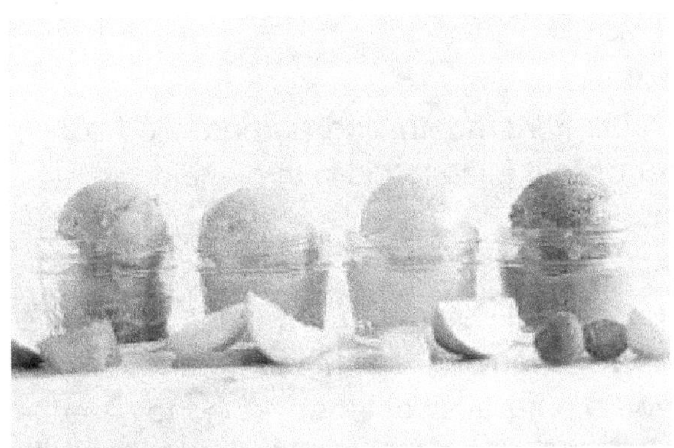

Ingredients:

- Fresh or frozen fruit (such as berries, mango, pineapple, peaches, etc.)
- Sweetener (honey, maple syrup, agave, etc.), optional
- Lemon or lime juice (for taste and to avoid browning)
- Water or fruit juice (if required for mixing)
- Optional add-ins (mint leaves, vanilla extract, etc.)

Instructions:

1. Prepare the Fruit:
   - Wash, peel (if required), and slice the fruit into tiny pieces.

2. Blend the Fruit:
   - Place the chopped fruit in a blender or food processor. If using frozen fruit, you may skip the chopping stage.

- Add a splash of lemon or lime juice to improve the taste and prevent the fruit from browning.

3. **Blend Until Smooth:**
   - Blend the fruit until it's smooth and pureed. Add a tiny quantity of water or fruit juice to aid with blending.

4. **Sweeten to Taste:**
   - Taste the fruit puree and determine whether you want to add a sweetener. Depending on the sweetness of the fruit, you may add a natural sweetener like honey, maple syrup, or agave. Start with a tiny quantity and adjust to taste.

5. **Add Optional Flavorings:**
   - Add flavourings, such as a dash of vanilla essence or a few fresh mint leaves, for a refreshing touch.

6. **Chill the Mixture:**
   - Place the fruit mixture in the refrigerator for approximately an hour to cool. This will help the sorbet freeze more evenly.

7. **Freeze:**
   - Pour the cooled fruit mixture into a shallow, freezer-safe container.

8. **Stir and Freeze:**

   - After around 30-45 minutes, take the container from the freezer and use a fork to stir the mixture. This will help break up any ice crystals and provide a smoother texture.

9. **Repeat Stirring:**

   - Repeat the stirring procedure every 30-45 minutes for several hours until the sorbet achieves a smooth and scoopable consistency.

10. **Serve:**

    - Once the sorbet is finished, scoop it into bowls or cones and enjoy your handmade fruit sorbet!

Homemade fruit sorbet is a light and refreshing treat that preserves fruit's natural taste. It's a healthier alternative to store-bought sorbets that typically include extra sugars and artificial additives. Experiment with various fruit combinations and enjoy a guilt-free frozen treat that's excellent for hot days or whenever you need something sweet and refreshing.

Coconut Date Bars

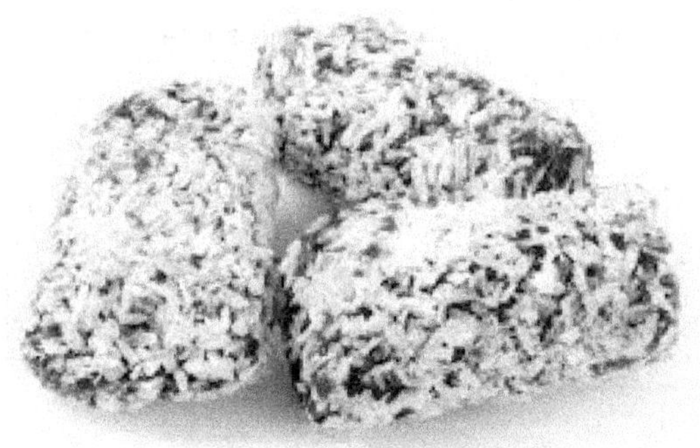

Ingredients:

- Medjool dates (pitted)
- Unsweetened shredded coconut
- Nuts (such as almonds, cashews, or walnuts)
- Nut butter (almond butter, peanut butter, etc.)
- Vanilla extract (optional)
- Pinch of salt (optional)
- Optional add-ins (chocolate chips, dried fruit, chia seeds, etc.)

Instructions:

1. **Blend Dates and Nuts:**
   - In a food processor, mix pitted dates and nuts. Pulse until the mixture creates a sticky and crumbly texture.

2. **Add Coconut and Nut Butter:**
   - Add unsweetened shredded coconut and a teaspoon of nut butter to the mixture.

3. **Flavor and Mix:**
   - Add a splash of vanilla essence and a dash of salt for taste if desired. Mix everything in the food processor until thoroughly mixed.

4. **Add Optional Add-Ins:**
   - Mix extra add-ins like chocolate chips, dried fruit, or chia seeds to increase texture and taste.

5. **Press into a Pan:**
   - Line a square or rectangular pan with parchment paper for easy removal.
   - Transfer the mixture to the pan and push it hard to form an equal coating.

6. **Chill:**
   - Place the pan in the refrigerator for an hour to firm up.

7. **Cut into Bars:**
   - Once the mixture has set, take it from the refrigerator and pull the parchment paper to remove the block from the pan easily.
   - Use a sharp knife to cut the block into bars of your preferred size.

8. Serve and Store:

- Coconut date bars are ready to be savoured! You may keep them in an airtight jar in the refrigerator for freshness.

9. Grab and Go:

- These bars make for a simple on-the-go snack or a healthy dessert choice.

Coconut date bars contain natural sweetness, fibre, and healthy fats. They're a terrific energy source and make for a delightful snack that may keep you powered throughout the day. Customize the recipe using your favourite nuts, nut butter, and add-ins to create a taste combination you enjoy.

Banana Oat Cookies

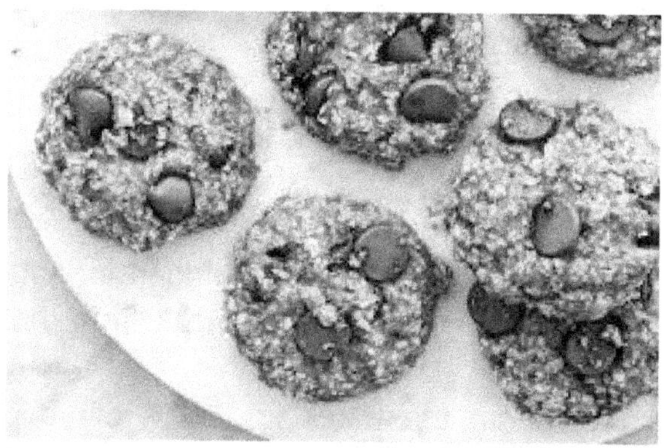

Ingredients:

- Ripe bananas (mashed)

- Rolled oats (old-fashioned oats)
- Optional add-ins (chocolate chips, raisins, almonds, cinnamon, vanilla essence, etc.)

Instructions:

1. Preheat the Oven:
   - Preheat your oven to 350°F (175°C) and line a baking sheet with parchment paper.

2. Mash Bananas:
   - In a mixing basin, mash ripe bananas until they are smooth and lumps-free.

3. Add Rolled Oats:
   - Add rolled oats to the mashed bananas. The ratio of mashed bananas to oats is typically approximately 2:1, but you may modify the quantity depending on the desired smoothness.

4. Mix and Add-Ins:
   - Mix the mashed bananas and oats until thoroughly blended. This will create the basis of your cookie dough.
   - If preferred, add optional add-ins such as chocolate chips, raisins, chopped almonds, a sprinkling of cinnamon, or a dash of vanilla essence for taste.

5. Drop Cookies on the Baking Sheet:
   - Use a spoon or cookie scoop to place spoonfuls of the cookie dough onto the prepared baking sheet. These

cookies don't expand much after baking, so you may shape them as desired.

6. **Bake:**
   - Bake the cookies in the oven for approximately 10-15 minutes or until they are firm and gently brown on the edges.

7. **Cool and Enjoy:**
   - Once cooked, remove the cookies from the oven and allow them to cool on the baking sheet for a few minutes.
   - Transfer the cookies to a wire rack to cool fully before consuming.

Store:
   - Store any leftover banana oat cookies in an airtight jar at room temperature or the refrigerator.

Banana oat cookies are a healthier alternative to typical cookies since they include no added sugars and are prepared with pure, natural ingredients. They are inherently gluten-free if you use certified gluten-free oats. These cookies are a terrific way to use ripe bananas and create a fast and gratifying snack that's excellent for kids and adults alike.

Nut Butter Stuffed Dates

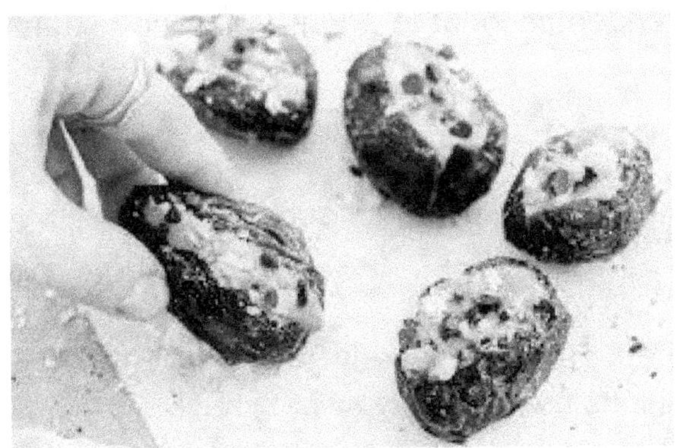

Ingredients:

- Medjool dates (pitted)
- Nut butter of your choosing (almond butter, peanut butter, cashew butter, etc.)
- Optional toppings (chopped almonds, cocoa powder, shredded coconut, etc.)

Instructions:

1. Prepare Dates:
   - Gently slice each pitted date along one side to create an aperture.

2. Add Nut Butter:
   - Using a teaspoon or a piping bag, delicately fill each date with your choice of nut butter.
   - The quantity of nut butter will depend on the size of the date.

3. Optional Toppings:

- Roll the filled dates in chopped almonds, chocolate powder, or shredded coconut to add flavour and texture if preferred.

4. Serve:

- Place the filled dates on a platter or serving dish.

5. Enjoy:

- Nut butter-stuffed dates are ready to be eaten! They make for a delicious and naturally sweet snack.

Nut butter-stuffed dates provide a delightful blend of natural sweetness, healthy fats, and protein. Medjool dates are naturally rich in fibre and vitamins, while nut butter gives satiety and taste. This snack is great for appeasing your sweet flavour while also delivering sustenance. Customize the flavours by combining various kinds of nut butter and toppings to create a range of tasty combinations.

CHAPTER NINE

Weekly Meal Plans

Here's an example weekly meal plan focusing on adrenal health by integrating balanced meals rich in nutrients and natural foods. Change portion amounts and ingredients depending on your tastes and dietary requirements.

Day 1: Monday

- **Breakfast:** Chia seed pudding topped with mixed berries and chopped almonds.
- **Lunch:** Grilled chicken salad with mixed greens, avocado, cherry tomatoes, and a lemon vinaigrette.
- **Snack:** Carrot sticks with hummus.
- **Dinner:** Baked salmon with quinoa and roasted Brussels sprouts.

Day 2: Tuesday

- **Breakfast:** Greek yoghurt parfait with sliced bananas, granola, and a sprinkle of honey.
- **Lunch:** Lentil and vegetable curry with brown rice.
- **Snack:** Handful of mixed nuts.
- **Dinner:** Zucchini noodles with tomato sauce and grilled chicken.

Day 3: Wednesday

- **Breakfast:** Nut butter banana pancakes topped with mixed berries.
- **Lunch:** Chickpea and vegetable stir-fry.
- **Snack:** Apple slices with almond butter.
- **Dinner:** Turkey or chicken wraps with whole-grain tortillas, mixed vegetables, and hummus.

Day 4: Thursday

- **Breakfast:** Oatmeal energy pieces and a side of mixed berries.
- **Lunch:** Black bean and sweet potato burrito dish with quinoa and avocado.
- **Snack:** Greek yoghurt with a sprinkling of cinnamon.
- **Dinner:** Grilled veggie quinoa dish with a tahini dressing.

Day 5: Friday

- **Breakfast:** Scrambled eggs with spinach and mushrooms.
- **Lunch:** Mediterranean chickpea salad with feta cheese.
- **Snack:** Cottage cheese with sliced peaches.
- **Dinner:** Vegetable stir-fry with tofu over brown rice.

Day 6: Saturday

- **Breakfast:** Whole-grain bread topped with avocado and a poached egg.
- **Lunch:** Tuna salad lettuce wraps with a side salad.
- **Snack:** Mixed berries with a handful of almonds.

- **Dinner:** Baked cod with roasted sweet potatoes and mixed greens.

Day 7: Sunday
- **Breakfast:** Coconut chia pudding with fresh mango.
- **Lunch:** Quinoa and black bean dish with avocado and salsa.
- **Snack:** Hummus with vegetable sticks.
- **Dinner:** Stuffed bell peppers with lean ground turkey and a side salad.

Remember that hydration is vital for adrenal health, so drink lots of water throughout the day. Listen to your body's hunger and fullness signals and alter portion sizes as appropriate. This meal plan emphasizes whole, nutrient-dense meals and attempts to deliver a range of nutrients to enhance general well-being and adrenal function.

CHAPTER TEN

Lifestyle Tips for Adrenal Health

Maintaining a healthy lifestyle is essential for supporting adrenal health and overall well-being. Here are some lifestyle habits that might assist in supporting good adrenal function:

1. **Prioritize Quality Sleep:** Aim for 7-9 hours of sleep every night. Establish a regular sleep schedule, create a calming bedtime routine, and ensure your sleep environment is conducive to rest.

2. **Manage Stress:** Practice stress management strategies such as deep breathing, meditation, yoga, or mindfulness. Regular relaxation may lessen the effect of chronic stress on your adrenal glands.

3. **Balanced Nutrition:** Consume a balanced diet rich in whole foods, including lean proteins, complex carbs, healthy fats, and various fruits and vegetables. Avoid excessive coffee, refined sweets, and processed meals.

4. **Stay Hydrated:** Drink lots of water throughout the day to maintain hydration. Herbal teas and infused water may also be hydrating solutions.

5. **Frequent Physical Activity:** Regularly exercise that meets your fitness level and preferences. Incorporate a

mix of aerobic activities, strength training, and flexibility exercises.

6. **Mindful Eating:** Pay attention to your body's hunger and fullness signs. Eat thoughtfully and avoid missing meals since irregular eating habits may stress the body.

7. **Restrict caffeine consumption:** Reduce or restrict caffeine consumption, particularly in the afternoon and evening, since much caffeine may interrupt sleep and stress the adrenals.

8. **Practice Time Management:** Organize your daily responsibilities and obligations to prevent overexertion and burnout. Prioritize tasks and delegate where required.

9. **Engage in Relaxation Activities:**
- Engage in hobbies you like.
- Spend time in nature.
- Practice deep breathing.
- Engage in activities that help you relax and unwind.

10. **Social Connections:** Foster meaningful social connections with friends and family. Spending time with loved ones and participating in healthy social interactions helps relieve stress.

11. **Limit Screen Time:** Reduce exposure to screens, particularly before sleep. Blue light from displays may interfere with sleep quality.

12. **Practice Self-Compassion:** Be gentle to yourself and practice self-compassion. Avoid perfectionism and unreasonable expectations.

13. **Mind-Body activities:** Incorporate mind-body exercises such as meditation, tai chi, or progressive muscle relaxation to improve relaxation and equilibrium.

14. **Seek practitioner Support:** If you suffer persistent tiredness, stress, or other symptoms, contact a healthcare practitioner. They can assist in detecting any underlying abnormalities and advise on maintaining adrenal health.

Remember that everyone's requirements and answers are unique. Listening to your body and making modifications that work for you is vital. Adopting a comprehensive strategy that covers physical, mental, and emotional well-being is crucial to boosting adrenal health and overall vitality.

Sustainable Changes for Long-Term Wellbeing

Creating lasting improvements for long-term wellness entails adopting habits and practices that are practical, pleasurable, and doable over time. Here are some recommendations for making permanent changes to your general health and wellness:

1. **Start Small:** Begin with one or two minor adjustments. Trying to modify your whole lifestyle at once might be stressful and unsustainable.

2. **Set Clear objectives:** Define clear and realistic goals consistent with your beliefs and priorities. Make them quantifiable and time-bound to measure your success.

3. **Attention on Behavior Change:** Shift your attention from short-term results (such as weight reduction) to modifying habits that contribute to your wellness (such as regular exercise and a balanced diet).

4. **Build behaviours Gradually:** Introduce new behaviours gradually, allowing your mind and body to acclimate. It takes time for habits to become automatic.

5. **Make it Enjoyable:** Choose activities you love and meals you appreciate. When you understand what you're doing, you're more inclined to remain with it.

6. **Practice Consistency:** Consistency is crucial to building habits. Aim to exercise your selected behaviours frequently, even in modest increments.

7. **Prioritize Balance:** Strive for a balanced approach to well-being. This involves physical exercise, diet, sleep, stress management, and emotional well-being.

8. **Listen to Your Body:** Pay heed to your body's messages. Rest when required, eat when hungry, and participate in things that make you feel good.

9. **Stay Flexible:** Life is unpredictable. Adapt to changes and failures without becoming disheartened. Embrace flexibility in your approach.

10. **Mindful Eating:** Practice mindful eating by enjoying each mouthful, eating carefully, and paying attention to hunger and fullness signs.

11. **Stay Hydrated:** Make drinking water a habit. Carry a reusable water bottle and drink throughout the day.

12. **Limit Screen Time:** Set restrictions on screen time to allow room for other activities that contribute to your wellness.

13. **Practice Self-Care:** Engage in things that energize you, whether reading, bathing, spending time in nature or practising a passion.

14. **Connect Socially:** Nurture ties with friends and family. Social links contribute to emotional wellness.

15. **Celebrate Progress:** Celebrate your victories, no matter how minor. Positive praise might drive you to persevere.

16. **Seek Support:** Share your objectives with supportive friends, family, or a coach. Having a support system may keep you accountable.

17. **Educate Yourself:** Stay knowledgeable about health and wellness, but be cautious of information sources. Choose evidence-based recommendations.

18. **Practice Gratitude:** Cultivate a gratitude practice by noticing the good parts of your life. This may increase your mood and general wellness.

19. **Reflect and Adjust:** Regularly analyze your progress and make modifications as required. Be open to modifying your approach over time.

20. **Celebrate Non-Scale Victories:** Recognize and celebrate victories beyond weight or looks, such as higher energy, better sleep, or enhanced endurance.

Remember that wellness is a journey; the process is as essential as the destination. Sustainable improvements are about developing a lifestyle that promotes your health and happiness in the long term.